Topographical and Pathotopographical Medical Atlas of the Chest, Abdomen, Lumbar Region, and Retroperitoneal Space

Scrivener Publishing
100 Cummings Center, Suite 541J
Beverly, MA 01915-6106

Publishers at Scrivener
Martin Scrivener (martin@scrivenerpublishing.com)
Phillip Carmical (pcarmical@scrivenerpublishing.com)

Topographical and Pathotopographical Medical Atlas of the Chest, Abdomen, Lumbar Region, and Retroperitoneal Space

Z. M. Seagal

Scrivener Publishing

WILEY

This edition first published 2018 by John Wiley & Sons, Inc., 111 River Street, Hoboken, NJ 07030, USA and Scrivener Publishing LLC, 100 Cummings Center, Suite 541J, Beverly, MA 01915, USA

For more information about Scrivener publications please visit www.scrivenerpublishing.com.

Wiley Global Headquarters
111 River Street, Hoboken, NJ 07030, USA

For details of our global editorial offices, customer services, and more information about Wiley products visit us at www.wiley.com.

Library of Congress Cataloging-in-Publication Data

ISBN 978-1-11952-6-261

Cover image: Courtesy of Z. M. Zeagal
Cover design by Kris Hackerott

Set in size of 13pt and Minion Pro by Exeter Premedia Services Private Ltd., Chennai, India

10 9 8 7 6 5 4 3 2 1

Contents

Preface

Atlas of Human Topographical and Pathotopographical Anatomy

Chest, Abdomen, Lumbar Region and Retroperitoneal Space

The atlas presents the topographic and pathotopographic anatomy of a person (adult and child). Sections "chest", "abdomen", "lumbar region" and "retroperitoneal space" include layered topographic anatomy, variant, computer and MRI topography and pathotopographic anatomy. Surgical anatomy of congenital malformations includes funnel-shaped deformation of the chest, keeled chest, hernia, aplasia, fistula, etc. Individual and age differences, fascia and cell spaces, triangles and vascular-neural bundles, and collateral blood supply are presented in case of injury or occlusion of the main arteries. All the pictures are colorful and original. The atlas is written in accordance with the educational program of medical universities of the Russian Federation. The original graphs of logical structures are presented according to the sections of topography and congenital malformations. This allows an effective study of the subject.

The atlas is intended for students of General Medicine, Pediatrics and Dentistry faculties, as well as for interns, residents, postgraduate students and surgeons.

The Chest

Topographic Anatomy of the Chest

Chest borders. The chest walls (*paries thoracis*) and chest cavity (*cavum thoracis*) together compose the chest (*thorax*). The superior chest border runs along the upper edge of the clavicle and the manubrium of sternum, and on the back — along the horizontal line drawn through the spinous process of the 7th cervical vertebra. The lower border goes down obliquely from the xiphoid process along the costal arches and on the back along the 12th rib and the spinous process of the 12th thoracic vertebra. The muscular-fascial layer of the chest is presented at the back with the latissimus dorsi muscle, on the sides with the serratus anterior muscles, and in front with the major and minor pectoral muscles. External and internal intercostal muscles are located in the chest itself; the space between these muscles is filled with cellular tissue with intercostal arteries, veins and nerves. The superior chest aperture (*apertura thoracis superior*) is bounded by the posterior surface of the manubrium of the sternum, the inner edges of the first ribs and the first thoracic vertebra. The inferior chest aperture (*apertura* *thoracis inferior*) is bounded by the posterior surface of the xiphoid process, the lower margins of the costal arches and the 10th thoracic vertebra anteriorly.

The prethoracic, thoracic, inframammary, scapular, subscapular and vertebral regions are identified.

Chest Cavity Organs Projection and Layers of Chest

Pleura projection (Figure 1). Lower pleural margins go on the midclavicular line — along the 7th rib; on the anterior axillary line — along the 8th rib; on the midaxillary line — along the 10th rib; on the scapular line — along the 11th rib; on the paraspinal line — until the 12th thoracic vertebra. Posterior margins correspond to costovertebral joints. The cervical pleura overhang the collar bone and correspond to the level of the spinous process of the 7th clervical vertebra posteriorly and anteriorly it is projected 2-3 cm above the collar bone.

Lung projection (Figure 2). The anterior margin of the left lung starts from the 4th costal cartilage. Then, because of the cardiac notch, it slants to the left midclavicular line. The lower margins of the lungs correspond to the 6th costal cartilage on the right sternal line and on the left parasternal line: on the midclavicular line — to the upper margin of the 7th rib; on the anterior axillary line — to the lower margin of the 7th rib; on the midaxillary line — to the 8th rib; on the scapular line — to the 10th rib, and on the parasinal line — to the 11th rib. The lung margin moves down in inhale. The lung apex is identified 3-4 cm above the collar bone.

Thymus (Figures 3, 4) is located in the superior interpleural space. Superiorly it borders on the jugular notch of the sternum, above the level of the 2nd rib; on the sides — with the parietal pleura margins.

Heart projection (Figure 5). Upper margin of the heart matches a horizontal line, drawn at the level of the 3rd costal cartilage insertion to the breast bone. The right margin is a line, connecting the upper edge

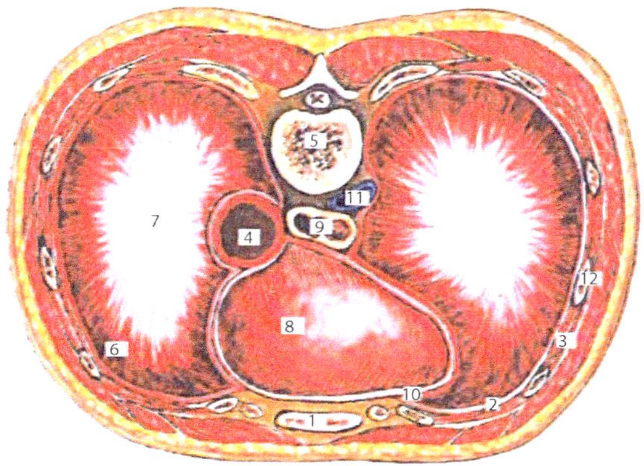

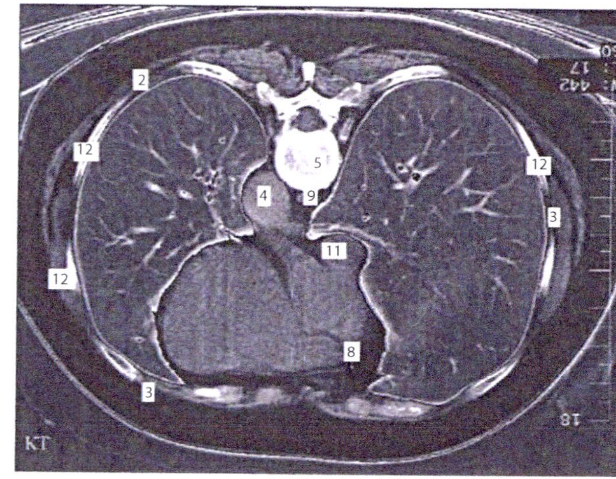

1 – breastbone;
2 – parietal pleura;
3 – intercostal muscles;
4 – aorta;
5 – vertebral body;
6 – costal part of diaphragm ;
7 – tendinous center of diaphragm;
8 – pericardium;;
9 – esophagus;
10 – costomediastinal sinus;
11 – inferior vena cava;
12 – ribs.

"he sintopia of the chest cavity organs is clearly visible on the computer tomogram: the inferior vena cava (11) and the esophagus (9) 0re located in front of backbone, to the right of which the aorta (4) is located, to which the heart with the pericardium (8) are attached.

Figure 1 Transverse section of the chest. Diaphragm.

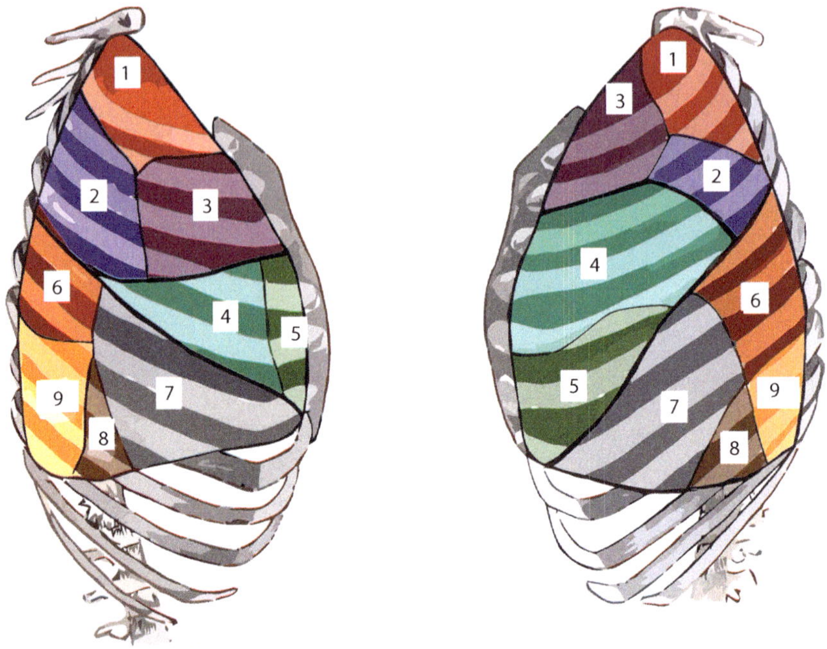

Figure 2 Lung segments.
Lobus superior: 1 – seg. apicale; 2 – seg. posterius; 3 – seg. anterius. Lobus medius: 4 – seg. laterale (правого легкого) et seg. lingulare superius (left lung); 5 – seg. mediale (right lung) et seg. lingulare inferius (left lung). Lobus inferior: 6 – seg. apicale; 7 – seg. basale anterius; 8 – seg. basale laterale; 9 – seg. basale posterius

of the 2nd rib on the right with the upper edge of the 3rd rib 1 cm to the right of the breast bone; then it continues in the form of the arch from the 3rd to the 5th ribs, as a bulge, heading to the right, at a distance of 1.5 cm from the right edge of the breast bone. The lower margin starts from the place where the 5th rib is attached on the right, through the metasternum base to the fifth intercostal space on the left, stopping short 1.5 cm from the midclavicular line.

The left margin is a line connecting the lower edge of the 1st rib on the left and the upper edge of the 2nd rib where they are attached to the breast bone, at the level of the 2nd intercostal space 2.5 cm to the left of the breast bone edge, then up to the point, placed 1.5-2 cm inwards the midclavicular line. The apex of the heart is projected on the left in the 5th intercostal space lower the 5th costal cartilage junction. An atrial

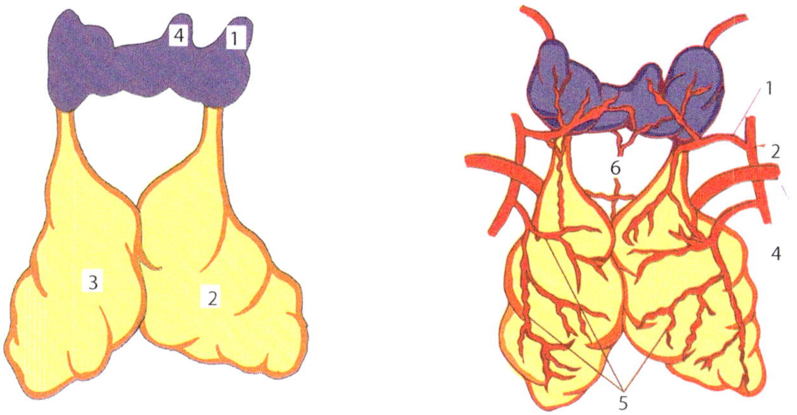

1 –lobus dexter gl. thyroideae; therocervicalis;

2 –lobus dexter thymi; thoracica interna;

3 –lobus sinister thymi;

6 –a. thyroidea ima

4 –istmus gl. thyroideae (lobus piramidalis)

Blood supply of thymus gland

1 –a. thyroidea inferior; 2 –truncus

3 –a. subclavia sinistra; 4 –a.

5 –rr. thymici a. thoracicae internae;

Figure 3 Thymus gland and its connection with the thyroid gland.

and ventrical borderline goes between the attachment points of the 3rd left and 6th right costal cartilages to the breast bone.

Thoracic aorta projection (Figure 6). The ascending aorta starts from the left ventricle at the level of the 3rd intercostal space behind the breast bone. It turns left and back, passing into the aortic arch at the level of the 2nd right sternocostal articulation.

Pulmonary trunk projection. The pulmonary artery starts from the right ventricle, left to the ascending aorta, in the 2nd intercostal space on the left.

Superior vena cava projection. The superior vena cava is formed by the confluence of two brachiocephalic veins at the level of the first costal cartilage attachment to the breast bone. It falls into the right atrium at the level of the 3rd costal cartilage.

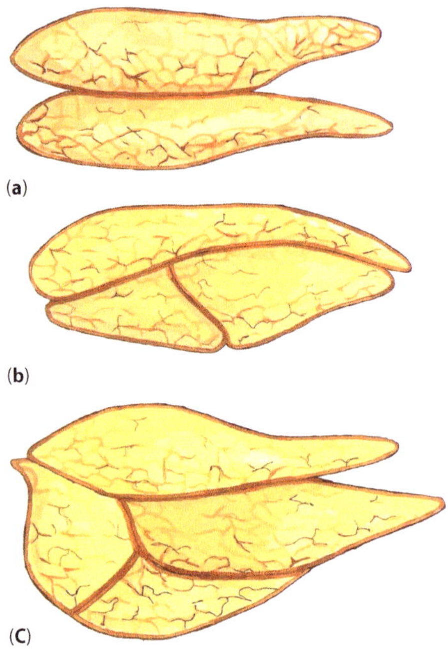

Figure 4 Differences in the shape and number of thymus glands.
a – two lobes, b – three lobes, c – four lobes.

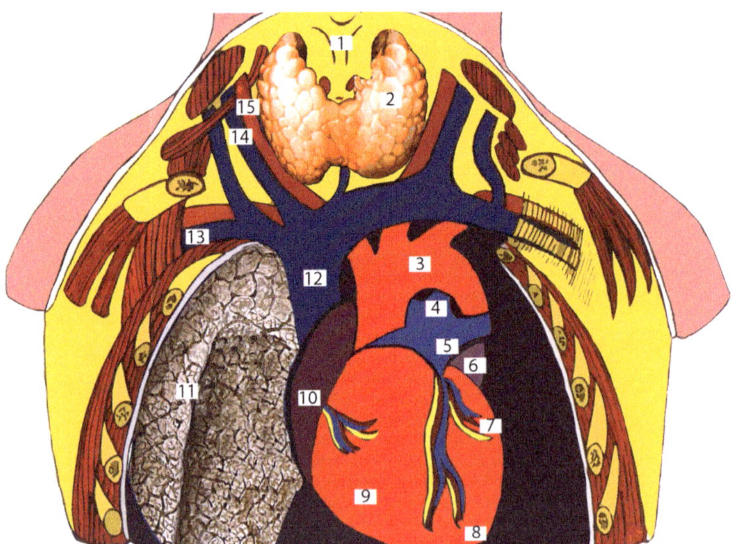

Figure 5 Topography of blood vessels, heart, right lung.
1 – larynx; 2 – gl. thyroidea; 3 – arcus aortae; 4 – truncus arteriosus; 5 – truncus pulmonalis; 6 – auricula sinistra; 7 – ventriculus sinister; 8 – apex cordis; 9 – ventriculus dexter; 10 – atrium dextrum; 11 – pulmo dextrum; 12 – v. cava superior; 13 – v. subclavia dextra; 14 – v. jugularis interna; 15 – a. carotis communis dextra.

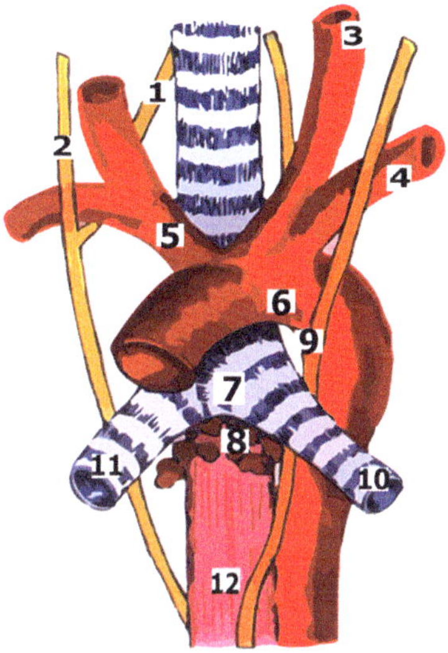

1 – n. recurrensdexter;
2 – n. vagus;
3 – a. carotiscommunis;
4 – a. subclavia;
5 – truncusbrachiocephalicus;
6 – arcusaortae;
7 – bifurcatiotracheae;
8 – nodilimphaticitracheobronchiales;
9 – n. recurrens sinister;
10 – bronchus sinister;
11 – bronchusdexter;
12 – oesophagus

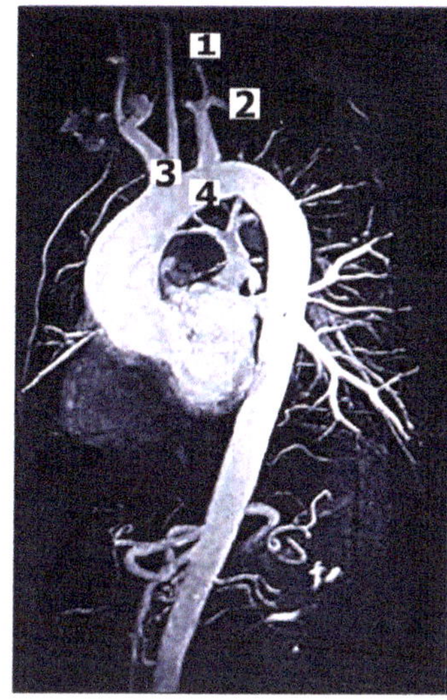

Топографияаорты
1 – общаясоннаяартерия;
2 – подключичная артер
3 – плечеголовной ствол;
4 – дугааорты

Figure 6 The relationship of the trachea, esophagus and aorta. Topography of the aorta.

Esophagus projection. The thoracic esophagus stretches from the superior thoracic aperture at the level of the 2nd thoracic vertebra; then at the level of the 2nd–4th thoracic vertebra, it lies to the right of the median line. Below the thoracic esophagus it crosses the median line again, and at the level of the 10th thoracic vertebra it enters through the esophageal opening, positioning itself 2.5 cm to the left of the median line.

Chest wall layers (Figure 7):

1. Skin - *derma*;
2. Subcutaneous fat - *panniculus adiposus*;

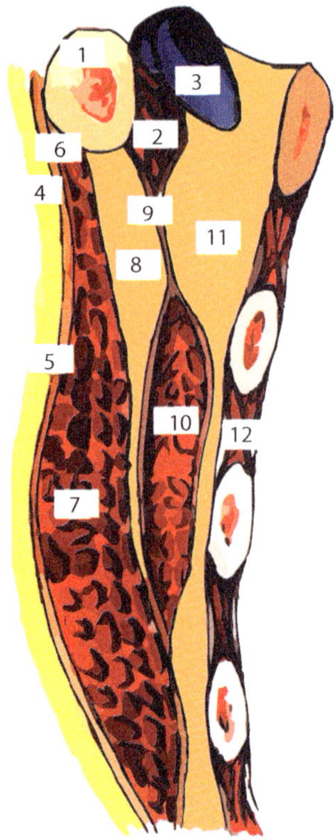

Figure 7 Layers of the front upper region of the sternum.
1 – clavicula; 2 – m. subclavicularis; 3 – v. subclavia; 4 – paniculus subdermalis; 5 – fascia superficialis; 6 – fascia propria; 7 – m. pectoralis major; 8 – spatium subpectorale superficialis; 9 – fascia coracoclaidocostalis; 10 – m. pectoralis minor; 11 – spatium subpectorale profundum; 12 – mm. intercostales

3. Subcutaneous veins
4. Suphenous nerves
5. Superficial pectoral fascia - *fascia pectoralis superficialis*;
6. Pectoral fascia - *fascia pectoralis propria*;
7. Major and minor pectoral muscles - *mm. pectoralis major et minor;*
8. Coracoclavicular pectoral fascia - *fascia coracoclavipectoralis*;
9. Endothoracic fascia - *fascia endothoracica.*

Vessels and nerves of the thoracic wall (Figures 8, 9) are divided into superficial and deep ones. Cutaneous branches of intercostal

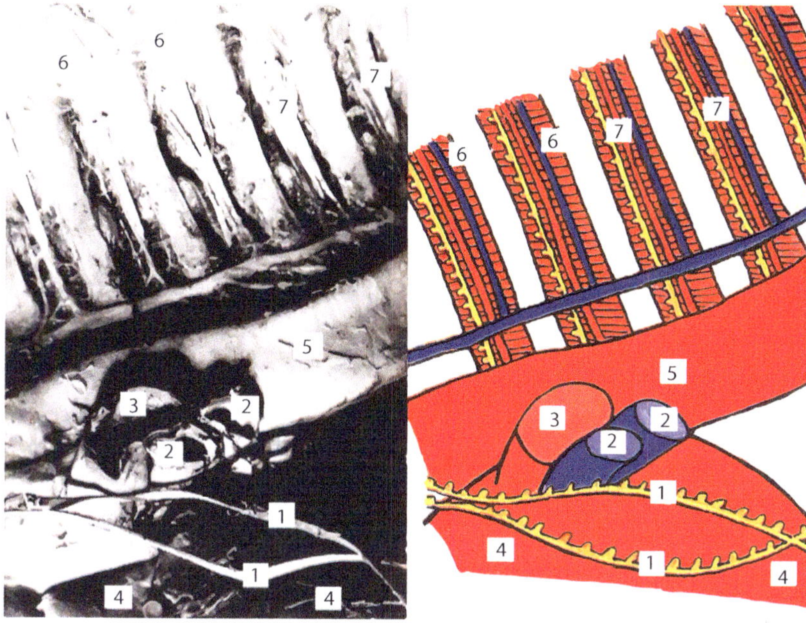

Figure 8 Vessels and nerves of the chest wall.
1 – n. vagus; 2 – vv. pulmonales; 3 – a. pulmonalis; 4 – cor; 5 – aorta; 6 – mm. intercostalis internii; 7 – a. intercostalis posterior et n. intercostalis

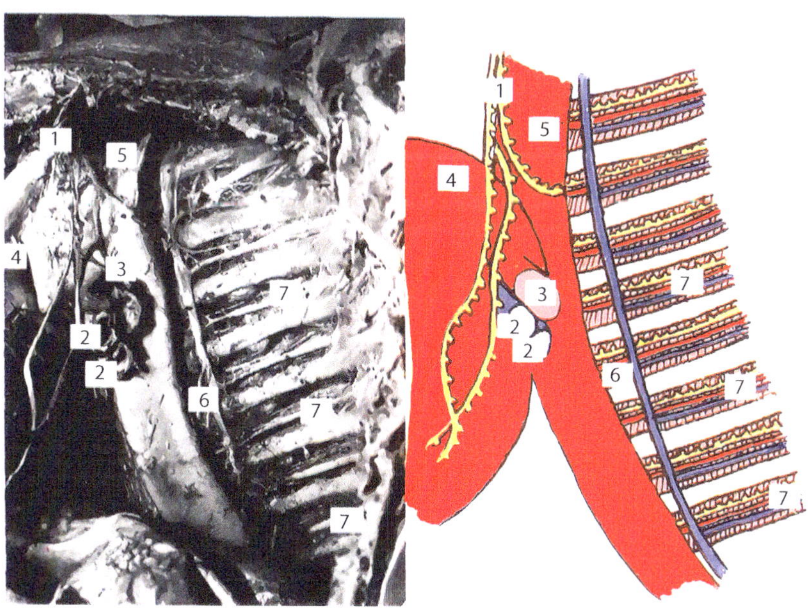

Figure 9 Vessels and nerves of the chest wall.
1 – n. vagus sinistra; 2 – vv. pulmonales; 3 – a. pulmonalis; 4 – cor; 5 – aorta; 6 – mm. intercostales; 7 – fasciculus vasus intercostalis

arteries—*a. thoracica interna, a. thoracica lateralis*—belong to superficial vessels. Superficial nerves branch from intercostal nerves, forming anterior and lateral cutaneous branches.

Arteries, including *a.thoracoacromialis, a. thoracica lateralis, a. thoracodorsalis, aa. Intercostales* and their branches belong to deep vessels. Deep layer nerves are presented by intercostal nerves producing muscular branches to intercostal muscles. The long thoracic nerve (*n. thoracicus longus*) goes down along the lateral surface of the serratus anterior. Anterior thoracic nerves come out of the infraclavicular triangle, previously perforating *fascia coracoclavipectoralis.*

There is also a fusiform cellular space around the esophagus. Intercostal spaces are spaces between exterior and interior intercostal muscles with *v. intercostalis posterior, a. intercostalis posterior,* and *n. intercostalis* placed downwards inside the intermucsular cell space of the intercostal space (Figure 10).

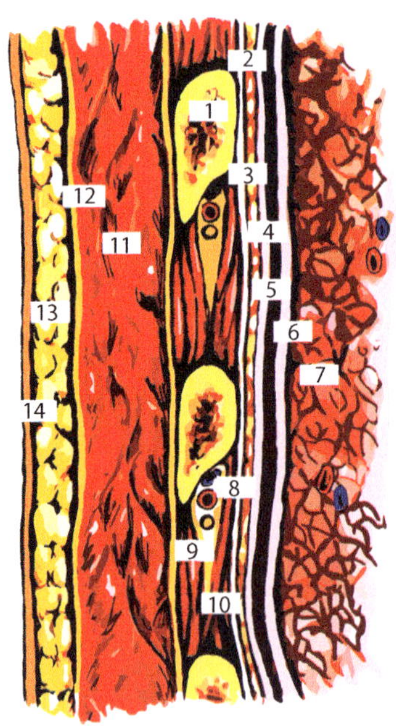

Figure 10 Intercostal space.
1 – costa; 2 – paniculus prepleuralis; 3 – fascia intercostalis; 4 – pleura parietalis; 5 – cavitas pleuralis; 6 – pleura visceralis; 7 – pulmo; 8 – v., a., n. intercostalis; 9 – m. intercostalis externus; 10 – m. intercostalis internus; 11 – m. pectoralis major; 12 – fascia sternalis; 13 – paniculus subdermalis; 14 – derma.

Mammary gland (Figures 11, 12). The female breast (*mamma muliebris)* differs depending on the age and individual anatomy.

It is placed on the anterior thoracic wall at the level from the 3rd to the 6th ribs.

The mammary gland reaches the breast bone medially; and laterally it goes down from the major pectoral muscle to the lateral chest wall, covering *m. serratus anterior*. There is an areola (*areola mammae)* in the middle part of the gland prominence, which has a nipple (*papilla mammae*) in its centre. The mammary gland is divided into four quadrants – upper outer, upper inner, lower outer, and lower inner. Between both mammary glands there is a deepening that is called a sinus (*sinus mammarum*).

The principal part of the breast (*corpus mammae*) consists of 15–20 lobes (*lobi mammae*); each of them has an excretory lactiferous

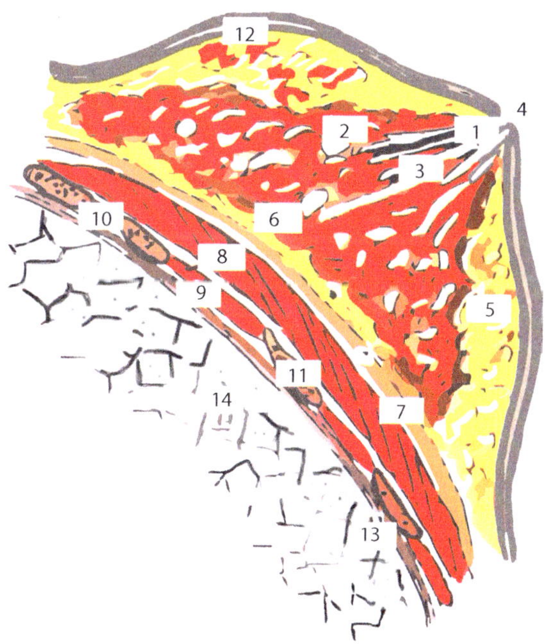

Figure 11 Mammary gland.
1 – sinus lactiferus; 2 – lobi gl. mammariae; 3 – ductus lactiferous; 4 – papilla; 5 – fatty tissue and interlobular connective tissue; 6 – cellular tissue between the superficial and own fascia; 7 – fascia pectoralis propria; 8 – m. pectoralis major; 9 – intercostal spaces; 10 – fascia intrathoracica; 11 – costa; 12 – fascia superficialis; 13 – pleura; 14 – pulmo.

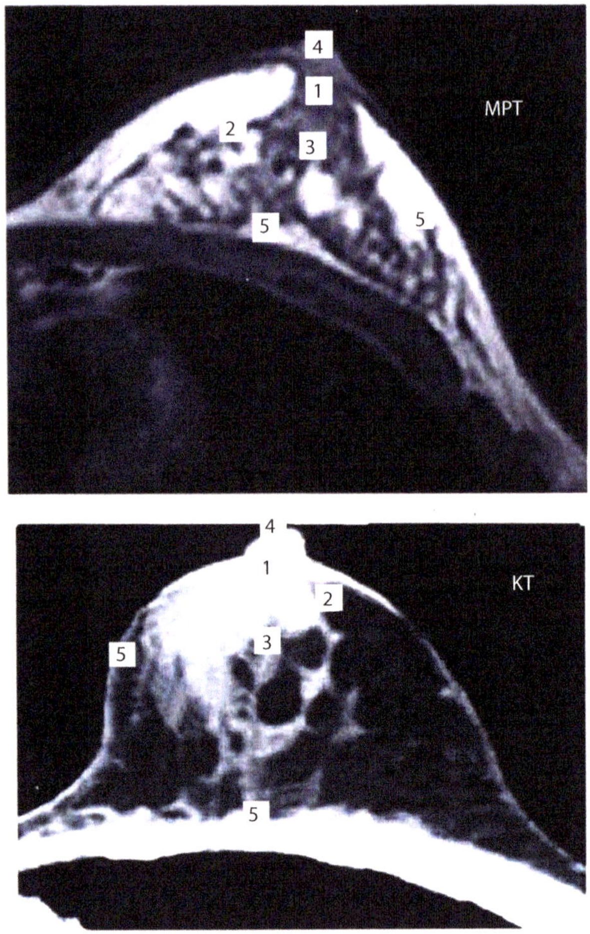

Figure 12 MRI and CT of the breast.
1 – milky sinus; 2 – lobules of the gland; 3 – milk ducts; 4 – thoracic nipple; 5 – thoracic fascia

duct (*ductus lactiferous*). Every 2–3 ducts merge and open with a lactiferous duct opening (*porus lactiferous*). A nipple may be of three different forms – cylindric, bulb-shaped, and conic.

Lactiferous ducts are opened directly on the tip of the nipple or inside the nipple. The common lactiferous sinus (*sinus lactiferous communis*) is formed from several merging lactiferous sinuses (*sinus lactiferous*).

The skin of the nipples and areola contains oil glands (*glandulae sebaceae*), perspiratory glands, (*glandulae sudorifera*), and special rudimentary lacteal glands (*glandulae areolares*).

Mammary gland blood supply is carried out from three sources: 1) internal thoracic artery (*a. thoracica interna*) that sends perforating branches (*rami perforantes*) to the 3rd – 5th intercostal spaces, which penetrate into mammary gland materia by the greater pectoral muscle perforation. 2) lateral thoracic artery (*a. thoracica lateralis*) that goes down along *m. serratus anterior* and springs frontwards the branches supplying external parts of the mammary gland with blood. 3) intercostal arteries (*aa. intercostales*) -- 3–7 intercostal arteries spring branches for mammary gland blood supply. All arteries inosculate with each other and surround lobes and ducts. The venous outflow is carried out by the same-name veins accordingly.

Mammary gland lymphatic system consists of lymphatic vessels positioned in three levels:

1) subpapillar lymphatic plexus (*plexus lymphaticus subpapillaris*); 2) superficial areol plexus (*plexus areolaris superficialis*); 3) profound areol plexus (*plexus areolaris profundus*). The main way for lymph outflow from the mammary gland is an axillary one. According to topoanatomic character, the axillary lymph nodes can be divided into five groups: 1) Lateral axillary nodes; 2) Central axillary nodes; 3) Medial or pectoral; 4) Subscapular or dorsal; and 5) Apical lymph nodes.

Innervation. There are genuine gland nerves and cutaneous gland nerves. Innervation is performed by anterior branches of 2nd – 7th intercostal nerves. Anterior nerve branches at the posterior surface form a plexus, which springs nerves, comprising its own plexus.

Diaphragm (Figure 13). The midriff or diaphragm separates the thoracic cavity from the abdominal cavity. It is divided into two parts: muscular (*pars muscularis diaphragmaticus*) and the central tendon of diaphragm (*centrum tendineum*).

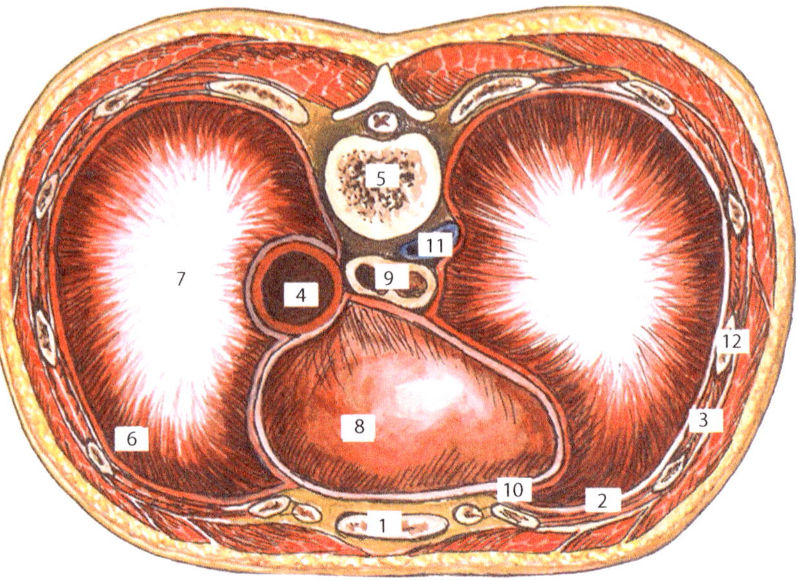

Figure 13 Diaphragm.
1 – sternum; 2 – pleura parietalis; 3 – mm. intercostales; 4 – aorta; 5 – corpus vertebrae; 6 – pars phrenicocostalis; 7 – centrum tendineum; 8 – pericardium; 9 – oesophagus; 10 – recessus costomediastinalis; 11 – v. cava inferior; 12 – costa.

The central tendon of diaphragm consists of the anterior folio (*folium anterius*) and lateral folios, (*folium dexter* and *folium sinister*) placed in the horizontal plane, and its muscular part— in vertical plane. The heart is placed at the anterior folio of the central tendon, and the lungs are placed at the lateral folios.

Depending on the attachment points, the muscular part of the diaphragm is divided into sternal part (*pars sternalis*), costal part (*pars costalis*), and lumbar part (*pars lumbalis*).

Diaphragm cruses of the lumbar part are the following:

1. *Crus mediale* – medial crus that starts from *lig. longitudinale anterius* and the body of the 3rd or 4th lumbar vertebra on the right; one vertebra higher on the left. Both cruses merge at the level of the 1st lumbar vertebra, restricting aortic hiatus for aorta and thoracic duct.

2. *Crus intermedius* – intermediate crus that starts from the lateral surface of the 2nd lumbar vertebra body and higher it passes into the muscular part of diaphragm.

3. *Crus laterale* – lateral crus that starts from the lateral surface of the 2nd lumbar vertebra forming two tendon arches and represents thickening *fascia endoabnominalis.*

Arcus lumbocostalis medialis—medial lumbocostal arch that starts from the 2nd lumbar vertebra body, bestrides *m. psoas major* and attaches to the transverse process of the 1st lumbar vertebra.

Arcus lumbo costalis lateralis – lateral lumbocostal arch starts from the transverse process of 1st lumbar vertebra, bestrides *m. quadratus lumborum* and attaches to the 12th rib.

Trigonum lumbocostale – lumbocostal triangle is placed between the lumbar and costal parts of diaphragm. It is based on the lower margin of the 12th rib. At the thoracic cavity side the triangle bottom is covered with pleura, adherent with thin fascial leaves, which are adjacent to kidneys and the posterior surface of adrenal capsule, surrounded with adipose capsule.

Trigonum sternocostale – sternocostal triangle is placed between sternal and costal parts of the diaphragm. Its height is from 1.8 to 2.7 cm; its base is from 2.5 to 3 cm.

The diaphragm has the following large apertures:

1. *Hiatus aorticus* — aortic hiatus — placed between medial cruses of diaphragm and their tendon part. Aorta and thoracic duct pass through the hiatus at the level of the 12th thoracic vertebra.

2. *Hiatus oesophageus* — esophageal hiatus; the medial crus of the diaphragm that twists after formation of the aortic hiatus, and then diverging again, forms the second hiatus

in the muscle part (*hiatus oesophageus*). The esophagus and the vagus nerve pass through it. The lumbar part of the diaphragm has two eight-shaped openings: a lower one – aortic (tendon) and upper one – esophageal (muscular).

3. *Foramen quadrilaterum s. venae cavae inferiori*—inferior vena cava quadrilateral foramen is placed in the right folio of the central tendon of diaphragm, where the inferior vena cava passes through.

Diaphragm blood supply (Figure 14). The anterior parts of the diaphragm periphery are supplied with blood by *aa. Intercostales* and its anterior part by *aa. pericardiacophrenicae* and *aa. intercostales.* Therefore, the system of descending aorta branches, thoracic and abdominal sections and subclavian artery take part in collateral circulation of diaphragm.

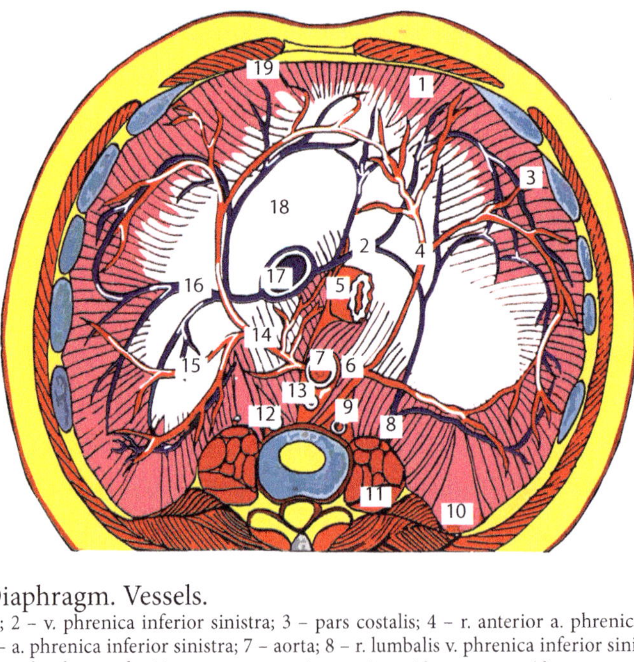

Figure 14 Diaphragm. Vessels.
1 – pars sternalis; 2 – v. phrenica inferior sinistra; 3 – pars costalis; 4 – r. anterior a. phrenica inferior sinistra; 5 – esophagus; 6 – a. phrenica inferior sinistra; 7 – aorta; 8 – r. lumbalis v. phrenica inferior sinistra; 9 – v. hemiazygos; 10 – trigonum lumbocostale; 11 – mm. psoas major et minor; 12 – v. azygos; 13 – truncus thoracicus; 14 – a. phrenica inferior dexera; 15 – rr. posteriors aa. phrenica inferior 16 – v. phrenica inferior dextra; 17 – v. cava inferior; 18 – centrum centrum tendineum; 19 – trigonum sternocostale

A. phrenica superior supplies the lumbar part of diaphragm as well as its pleura with blood from the thoracic cavity side. *A. phrenica inferior* supplies the diaphragm and abdominal membrane with blood; besides the left artery supplies terminal esophagus part, and the right one — the inferior vena cava wall, inferior diaphragm veins,

vv. phrenicae inferioris falls into the inferior vena cava, adhering by two to the same name artery.

Diaphragm innervation. Phrenic nerve (*N. Phrenicus*) outgoes from the anterior branches of the 3rd -4th cervical nerves. The left phrenic nerve penetrates the diaphragm and branches on its inferior surface, the right one ends with its branches on the superior surface of diaphragm. Six inferior intercostal nerves take part in the innervation of the posterior part of the diaphragm.

Surgical Anatomy of Thoracic Wall Congenital Malformation

Hollowed chest is a congenital malformation caused by hyperplasia of the inferior pair of ribs and their cartilages. The midsternum is retroposed and forms a deepening. The deformation is often asymmetric; the degree of manifestation varies heavily.

Keeled chest is a protruding deformation of the breast bone, which occurs more rarely than the hollowed chest.

Amastia is a fetal pathology resulting in the birth of a child without one or both mammary glands. In this case, breast feeding is impossible. Malformation may come with deficiencies of the ovary or other systems, which results in developmental disorder of the whole reproductive system. Such a woman has neither breast tissue nor nipple.

Polymastia is the presence of additional, multiple glands and nipples, appearing as developed or underdeveloped glands, with clear nipples, placed along “the milk line”, which passes from the axillary cavity to the femoroinguinal area. Thereby, additional glands may swell and lactate while service period.

Gynekomastia is mammary gland enlargement in men with glands and fatty tissue hypertrophy. Painful asymmetric breast lumpiness often appears and then disappears spontaneously. The size of lumpiness may be different. Physiologic gynecomastia occurs in newborns, puberty and old men. There is also a pathologic form of gynecomastia.

Diaphragmatic hernia is an outpunching of the esophagus, stomach or small bowel through the diaphragm into the thoracic cavity. The work of the esophageal sphincter which closes the pass between esophagus and stomach is thereby disrupted.

Diaphragm aplasia is an abnormal development of the diaphragm, when a part of the diaphragm or a section of a part is absent. Newborns may have a congenitally missing diaphragm, which is fatal. One can distinguish between unilateral and total diaphragm aplasia. Unilateral aplasia may be full or partial.

Relaxation of diaphragm is cupula relaxation and high-position of the diaphragm, based on paralysis, drastic thinning and constant displacement of diaphragm into the thoracic cage together with adjacent abdominal cavity organs. The congenital elevation of the diaphragm is connected with aplasia or underdevelopment of its muscular part, and also with fetal trauma or aplasia of phrenic nerve. Acquired elevation appears because of secondary atrophy, phrenic nerve injury or diaphragm injury: trauma or tumor.

Thoracic Cavity

Pleura is the serosa of lungs divided into two layers: parietal pleura (*pleura parietalis*) and visceral pleura (*pleura viscerali*). The latter layer covers the pulmonary surface and forms the pulmonary ligament (*lig. pulmonale*) in the root of the lung area while passing into the parietal folium. It is placed under pulmonary veins and stretches vertically down almost to the inferior margin of the lung. A narrow stripe of the lung between pulmonary ligament layers is not covered with the visceral layer of pleura.

Parietal pleura are subdivided into several sections:

1. *Pleura costalis* – costal pleura that covers the internal surface of the thoracic cage and is firmly adhered to endothoracic fascia (*fascia endothoracica*).

2. *Cupula pleurae* – cupula of the pleura that outstands over the first rib, entering the neck area. On the back, the cupula of pleura apex is placed at the level of the neck of the 1st rib, and at the front (anterior) it is placed 2-3 cm above the collar bone. On the top, in the anterior area, the subclavian artery is attached to the cupula of pleura. The artery leaves a mark on the serous folio – sulcus of subclavian artery (*sulcusa. Subclaviae*).

3. *Pleura diaphragmatica* – diaphragmal pleura that covers the superior surface of the cupula of the diaphragm without touching the area of anterior folio (*folium anterior*) of the diaphragm, which is accreted by the heart sac – pericard (*pericardium*).

4. *Pleura mediastinalis* – mediastinal pleura that serves as side walls of the mediastinum.

The pleural sinuses (*sinus pleurae*) are as follows:

1. *Sinus phrenicocostalis* – phrenocostal sinus – it is formed by transition of parietal diaphragmal pleura into the costal pleura. This sinus is particularly deep on the right and lies about 9 cm down along *linea axillaris dextra*.

2. *Sinus costomediastinalis anterior* – anterior costomediastinal sinus is placed between the anterior part of mediastinal and costal pleura. It is placed near the anterior margin of the lung where the costal surface of the lung transits into its mediastinal surface.

3. *Sinus costomediastinalis posterior* – posterior costomediastinal sinus that is placed on the back, where costal

pleura transits into mediastinal one. Both latter sinuses lie in a vertical direction.

4. *Sinus phrenicomediastinalis* – phrenomediastinal sinus is a narrow space, placed horizontally in sagital direction, where the diaphragm pleura transits into the mediastinal one.

The layers of the costal pleura separate at the suprasternal notch area, behind the presternum, forming the superior interpleural area (*area interpleurica superior*), where the thymus is placed. By separation of the costomediastinal sinuses, the inferior interpleural area (*area interpleurica inferior*) is formed downwards.

Lungs. Superior lobes. The superior margin of the lung lobes passes 3–4 cm above the collar bone.

On the back, it corresponds with the spinous process of the 7th cervical vertebra. The inferior margin is projected to the 5th rib along the paraspinal line, to the 4th–5th intercostal space along the scapular line, to the 4th–5th intercostal space along the midaxillary line, to the 5th rib along the mammary line.

The superior lobe of each lung has **three segments:** anterior, posterior and apical, the proximal bronchus has the same division. The anterior segment of the superior lobe by its anterior surface is attached to the internal surface of the anterior wall of the thoracic cage; the posterior segment fills the apical part of the cervical pleura, the apical segment — between and outside of them.

Middle lobes. The middle lobe of the lung (*lobus anterior*) is of triangular shape and placed at the anterior between the superior and inferior lobes. The anterior margin of the middle lobe is the inferior margin of the superior one. The inferior margin is identified along the scapular and midaxillary lines at the level of the 6th–7th intercostal space, along the mammary line at the level of the 6th rib. There are **two segments**: lateral and medial. The middle lobes do not reach the paraspinal line. The middle lobe of the left lung in its internal structure is close enough to the middle lobe of the right lung constitution. The superior surface of the left middle lobe is adherent with the inferior lobe. According to the lobar bronchus division, each of the middle lobes is divided into **three segments**: superior, middle and inferior.

Inferior lobes. The volume of the inferior lobe of each lung is significantly higher than the volumes of all other lobes. The inferior lobe is in the form of frustum. Each lobe consists of five segments: anterior, posterior, external, internal basalis, and apical.

Lung hilum (*hilus pulmonis*) is a part of the medial surface of lungs, where vessels, main bronchus and nerves pass through.

Roots of lungs. The root of lung consists of bronchus, pulmonary artery, two pulmonary veins, bronchial arteries and veins, lymph tubes and nerves. On the right, from top downward there is right bronchus; *ramus dexter a. pulmonalis* – right pulmonary artery; *vv. Pulmonales* – pulmonary veins. On the left, the highest position is occupied by *ramus sinister a. Pulmonalis* – left pulmonary artery; lower there is *bronchus sinister* – left bronchus, then pulmonary veins; (anatomical code for right lung – V, A, C; for left lung – A, B, V) (Figures 15, 16).

The right root of the lung is surrounded by the azygos vein (*v. azygos*) posteriorly and superiorly; by superior vena cava (*v.cava superior)* anteriorily; by inferior vena cava (*v.cava inferior)* inferiority; medially it is surrounded by the ascending aorta, laterally – by *n. phrenicus, a. pericardiacophrenica.* The left root of the lung is surrounded with an aortic arch superiorly; esophagus, vagus and thoracic aorta posteriorly; heart and pericardial sac anteriorly and inferiorly; medially – with the ascending aorta; laterally – with *n. phrenicus, a. Pericardiacophrenica.*

Structural features of pleura, pleural cavities and lungs of children. Due to the fact that the volume of lungs, especially for newborns, is small, the upper chest is narrower, and the lower chest is expanded due to the high position of the diaphragm and liver adhesion. It determines the form of chest that is constricted in the upper sections and expanded downwards. Gradually, it reshapes into the form of chest common for an adult.

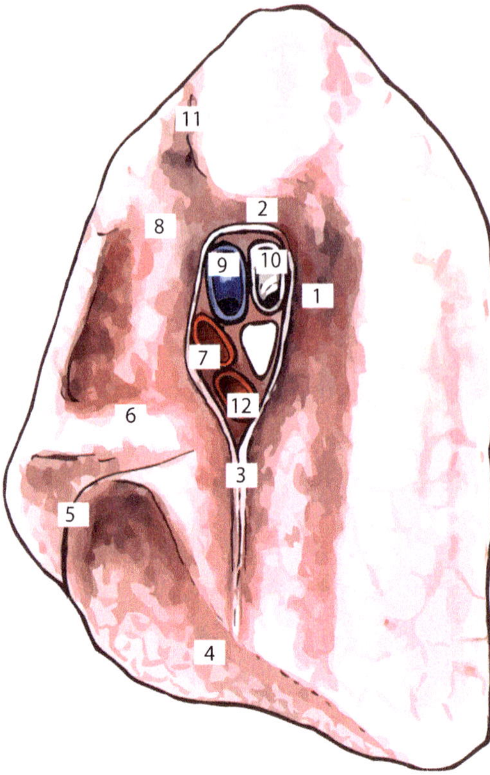

Figure 15 Right lung.
1 – impressio oesophagialis; 2 – impressio v. azygos; 3 – lig. pulmonalis; 4 – facies diaphragmatica; 5 – sulcus interlobares; 6 – fossa cardiaca; 7 – v. pulmonalis superior; 8 – impressio superior; 9 – a. pulmonalis; 10 – bronchus; 11 – impressio a. subclavia; 12 – v. pulmonalis inferior

The cupula of the pleura of a newborn is 0.5 cm above the 1st rib. With age due to the sinking of anterior parts of ribs, this part of pleura increases, and at the age of five the cupula of pleura outstands for 2–3 cm above the 1st rib.

In newborns and infants, the peculiarity of pleural layers is in their tenuity, unstable connection with peripleural tissue and displacement of parietal pleura with formation of relatively large extrapleural sections (superior and inferior). It happens due to the presence of a large size thymus in anterior mediastinum and transverse position of a child's heart.

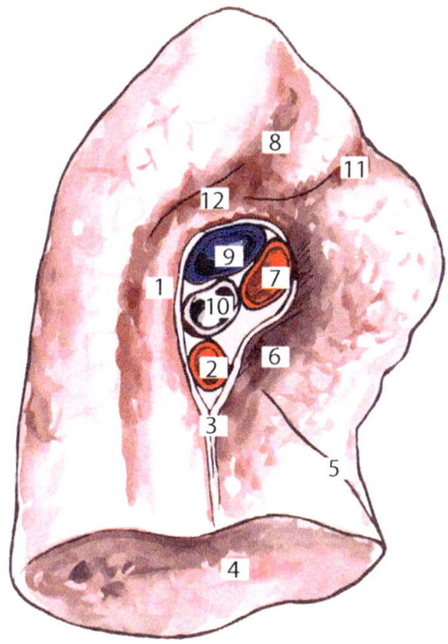

Figure 16 Left lung.
1 – impressio parties aortae descendens; 2 – v. pulmonalis inferior; 3 – lig. pulmonalis; 5 – sulcus interlobares; 6 – fossa cardiaca; 7 – v. pulmonalis superior; 8 – impressio a. communis; 9 – a. pulmonalis; 10 – bronchus sinister; 11 – impressio a. subclavia; 12 – impressio arcus aortae

Children's pleural sinuses are relatively deep. Because of the large thymus gland, one can mark out additional cove-shaped recessions of pleural cavities: sternothymic and pericardiothymic. With child development, the alignment of the pleural torsion happens together with restoration of the pulmonary tissue resulted from respiratory excursions.

Mediastinum Topography (Figures 17, 18, 19)

Mediastinum (*mediastinum*) is a space between internal surfaces of lungs, covered with pleura. It is divided into upper and lower floors (Figure 20).

All anatomic organizations lying above the superior margin of pericard belong to the superior mediastinum; the superior mediastinum is bounded by the thoracic inlet and the line drawn between Louis angle and intervertebral disc Th4-Th5.

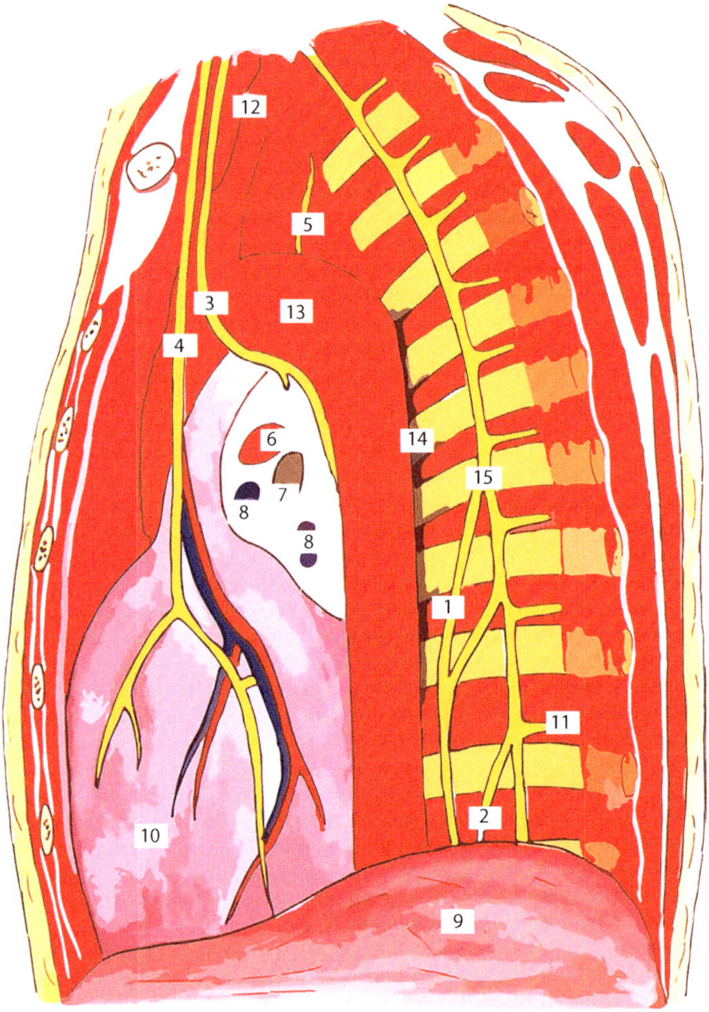

Figure 17 Posterior mediastinum, left view.
1 – n. splanchnicus major; 2 – n. splanchnicus minor; 3 – n. vagus; 4 – phrenic nerve and accompanying vessels; 5 – n. recurrens; 6 – a. pulmonalis; 7 - bronchus sinister; 8 – vv. pulmonales; 9 – diaphragma; 10 – pericardium; 11 – sympathetic branch to the intercostal nerves; 12 – a. subclavicularis; 13 – arcus aortae; 14 – v. hemiazigos; 15 – truncus simpaticus

The inferior mediastinum is bound by the upper margin of the pericard superiorly and by the diaphragm inferiorly. It is divided into anterior, medial and posterior areas.

Anterior mediastinum (Figure 21). The anterior mediastinum is bound by the breast bone anteriorly and by the pericard and brachiocephalic

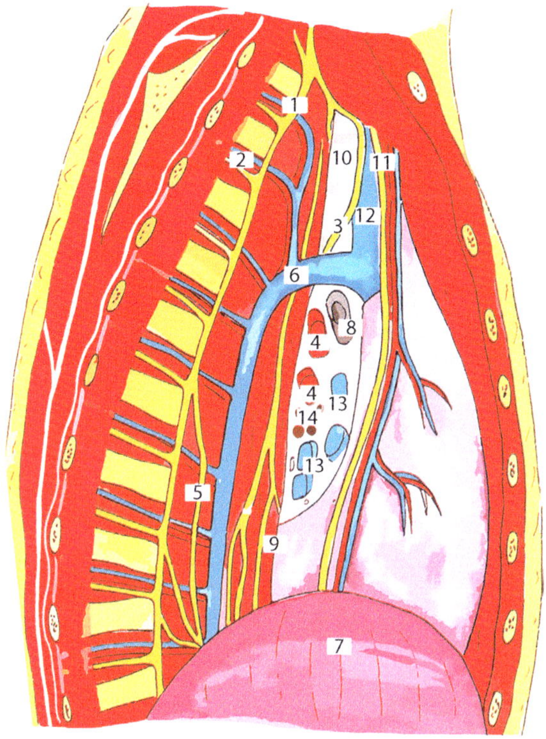

Figure 18 Posterior mediastinum, right view.
1 – truncus simpaticus; 2 – vv. et vases intercostales; 3 – n. vagus; 4 – a. pulmonalis; 5 - n. splanchnicus major; 6 – v. azygos; 7 – diaphragma; 8 – bronchus dexter; 9 – oesophagus; 10 – trachea; 11 – n. diaphragmaticus; 12 – v. cava superior; 13 – vv. pulmonales; 14 – nodi lymphatici.

vessels posteriorly. The heart with pericard, thymus, ascending aorta, aortic arch, arterial duct of main pulmonary artery, superior and inferior vena cava, pulmonary veins, and also phrenic nerves and vessels are placed in it.

Thymus gland (*glandula thymus*) is placed in *area interpleurica superior,* behind the manubrium of sternum. It is fully matured by the age of 2–3, and then the process of involution starts. Superiorly at some distance from thymus gland, there is a thyroid gland; inferiorly – the anterosuperior surface of heart sac; laterally it borders with the mediastinal pleura. The anterior mediastinal lymph nodes (*l-dimediastinales anteriores*) in number of 10–12 are placed anteriorly around the gland, buried in fatty tissue.

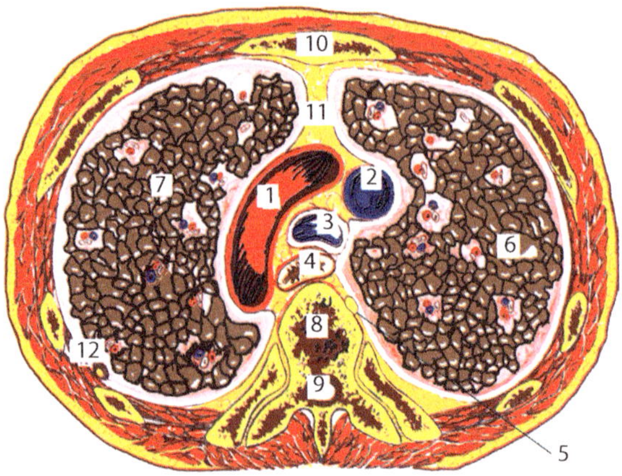

Figure 19 Transverse section of the breast.
1 – arcus aorte; 2 – v. cava superior; 3 – trachea; 4 – oesophagus; 5 - truncus simpaticus; 6 – pulmo dexter; 7 – pulmo sinister; 8 – vertebra; 9 – medulla spinalis; 10 – sternum; 11 – paniculus mediastini anterius; 12 – pleura.

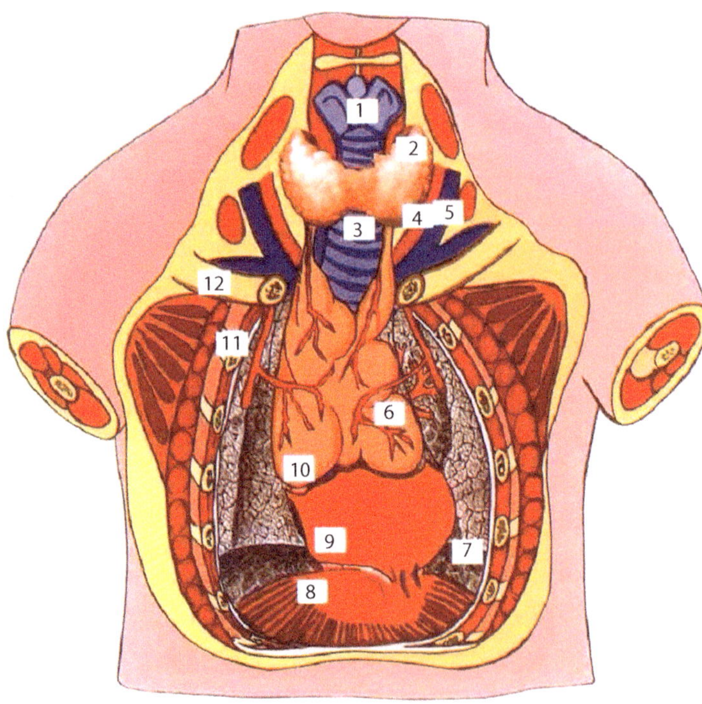

Figure 20 Organs of anterior mediastinum and neck.
1 – larynx; 2 – gl. thyroidea; 3 – trachea; 4 – a. carotis communis; 5 – v. jugularis interna; 6 – lobus sinister thymi; 7 – pulmo; 8 – diaphragma; 9 – pericardium; 10 – lobus dexter thymi; 11 – a. thoracica interna; 12 – clavicula.

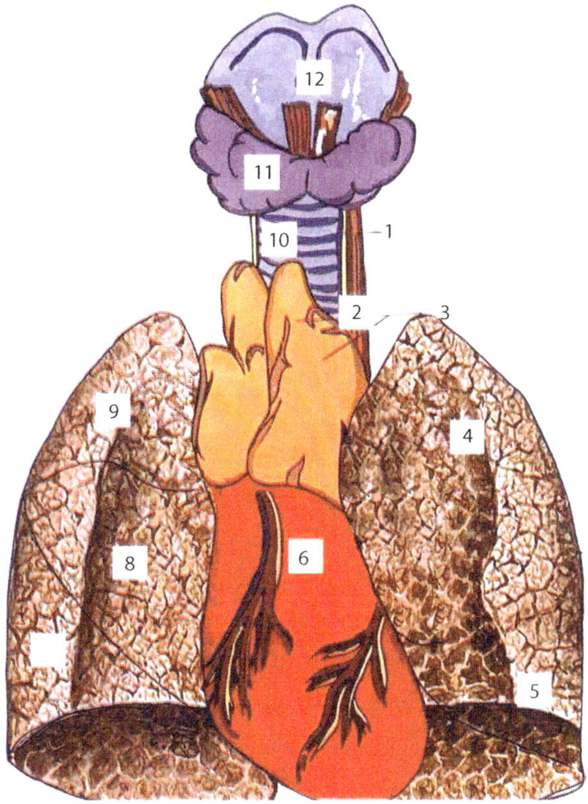

Figure 21 Syntopia of the chest cavityorgans and neck.
1 – n. laryngeus reccurens; 2 – esophagus; 3 – thymus; 4 – lobus superior pulmonis sinistri; 5 – lobus inferior pulmonis sinistri; 6 – cor; 7 – lobus inferior pulmonis dexter; 8 – lobus medius pulmonis dextri; 9 – lobus superior pulmonis dextri; 10 – trachea; 11 – gl. thyroidea; 12 – larynx

Pericard (*pericardium*) (Figure 22). The heart sac cavity (*cavum pericardii*) is in a form of cone, the base of which formed by its diaphragm surface (*facies diaphragmatica*) is placed inferiorly and adherent to the tendon part of the diaphragm. A gradually spiring vertex surrounds the primary segment of aorta.

The following parts of the heart sac are distinguished:

1. *Pars sternocostalis pericardii* – sternocostal part of the heart sac is faced forward and adjacent to the inferior part

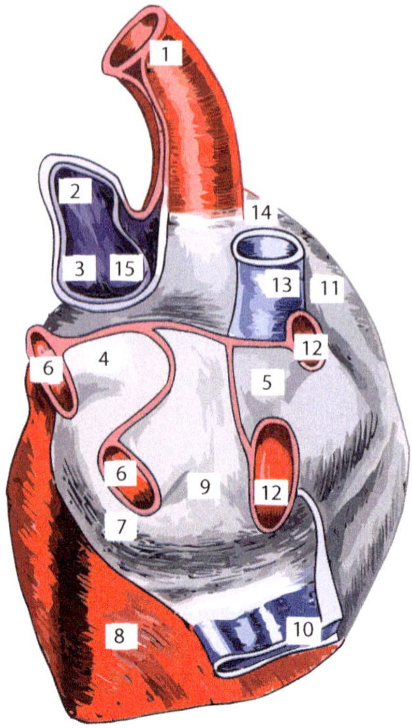

Figure 22 Infant's pericardium.
1 – aorta; 2 – ductus arteriosum; 3 – a. pulmonalis sinister; 4 – основание сумки перикарда перед венами; 5 – основание сумки перикарда за венами; 6 – vv. pulmonales sinistrae; 7 - atrium sinistrum; 8 – ventriculus sinister; 9 – sinus obliqus pericardii; 10 – v. cava inferior; 11 – atrium dextrum; 12 – vv. pulmonales dextrum; 13 – v. cava superior; 14 – sinus transversus pericardii; 15 – a. pulmonalis dextra.

of sternum body and to internal parts of the 4th–5th intercostal spaces.

2. *Partes mediastinales pericardii dextra et sinistra* – the right and left mediastinal parts of heart sac are placed on the sides of heart and border with mediastinal parts of pleura. Phrenic nerves (*nn. phrenici*) and pericardial abdominothoracic vessels (*vasa pericardiacophrenica*) are also placed here.

3. *Pars vertebralis pericardii* – the spinal part of the heart sac is reverted to the spine. The esophagus, azygos vein, thoracic duct and thoracic part of the aorta are adjacent to the posterior surface.

4. *Pars diaphragmatica* – the abdominothoracic surface of the heart sac is firmly accreted to the central tendon and partly to the muscular part of the diaphragm.

The heart sac is fixed in its position:

1. Diaphragmatic surface of the heart sac is firmly accreted to the tendon part of the diaphragm. The so- called heart bed is formed here.

2. Superiorly, the pericard is accreted to the aorta, pulmonary artery and superior vena cava.

3. Special ligament takes part in the heart sac fixing:
   a. *lig. sternocardiacum superius* – superior thoracicocardial ligament that goes from the manubrium of the sternum to the heart sac.

   b. *lig. sternocardiacum inferius* – inferior thoracicocardial ligament that goes between the posterior surface of metasternum and the anterior surface of the pericard.

The blood supply of the pericard is performed by the following vessels:

1. *a. pericardiacophrenica* – the pericardiacophrenic artery is a branch of *a. thoracica interna*, that goes along with *n. phrenicus* and branches off in the heart sac and diaphragm, supplying its anterior and lateral sides with blood.

2. *rami pericardiaci* – pericardial branches come directly from thoracic aorta, and supply the posterior wall of the pericard with blood.

Venous outflow is performed through pericardial veins, *vv. pericardiaci,* directly into the superior vena cava system.

The heart sac **innervation** is performed by nervules from the phrenic and vagus nerves, and sympathis branches from cardiac plexus.

Lymph outflow from the heart sac is performed into the following lymph nodes:

1. *L-di sternales* – sternal lymph nodes that are placed alongside of breastbone, along *vasa thoracica interna.*

2. *L-di mediastinales anteriores* – anterior mediastinal lymph nodes that are placed at the anterior surface of aortic arch.

3. *L-di phrenici anteriores* – anterior phrenic lymph nodes, the so-called anterior mediastinal lymph nodes, are bedded on the diaphragm at the level of the metasternum.

4. *L-di mediastinales posteriores* – posterior mediastinal lymph nodes collect lymph from the posterior wall of the pericard.

Lymph tubes from anterior and posterior mediastinal nodes reach the thoracic duct on the left and right lymphatic duct on the right.

Heart topography (Figures 23, 24, 25, 26). The heart, by its larger part, is placed in the left section of the thoracic cage within the limits of the anterior mediastinal. Laterally, it is bounded by the layers of mediastinal pleura. The third part of the heart is placed to the right of the median line and gets into the right section of the thoracic cage.

The superior margin of the heart passes along the 3rd costal cartilages. The inferior margin goes obliquely from the place where the 5th costal cartilage is attached to the fifth intercostal space of the left side. The right margin starts under the upper edge of the 3rd rib, 1.5–2 cm outward of the edge of breast bone, then it continues up to the place where the 5th costal cartilage is attached to the breast bone. The left margin

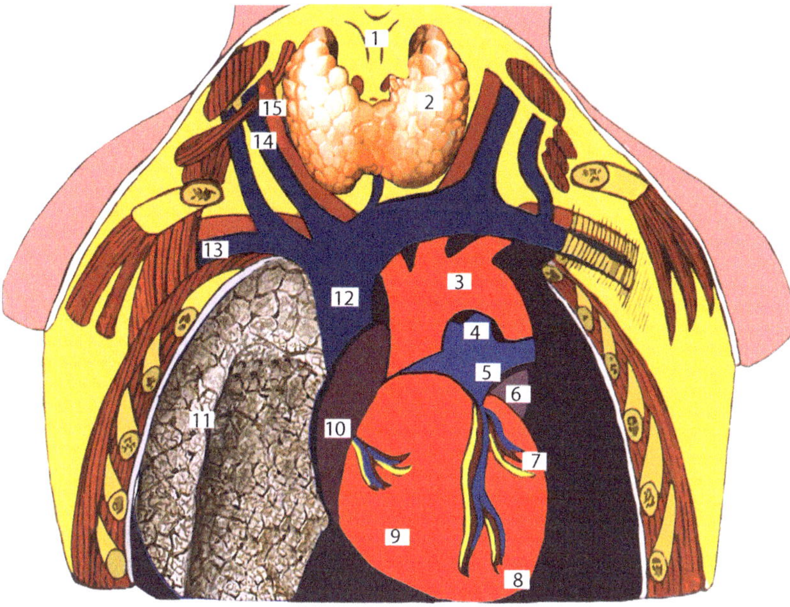

Figure 23 Topography of blood vessels, heart, right lung.
1 – larynx; 2 – gl. thyroidea; 3 – arcus arcus aortae; 4 – ductus arteriosus; 5 – truncus pulmonalis; 6 – aoricula sinister; 7 – ventriculus sinister; 8 – apex cordis; 9 – ventriculus dexter; 10 – atrium dextrum; 11 – pulmo dextrum; 12 – v. cava superior; 13 – v. subclsvia dextra; 14 – v. jugularis interna; 15 – a. carotis communis dextra

is bulgy, 3-3.5 cm outwards the edge of the breast bone, and inferiorly – 1.5 cm inwards the midclavicular line.

Heart syntopy (Figure 27). Anteriorly the heart is covered with mediastinal pleura layers. External compartments of the heart are covered up with lungs on both sides, filling anterior costomediastinal sinuses. At the back, organs of posterior mediastinal are attached to the heart: the esophagus with vagus nerves, thoracic aorta, on the right – azygos vein, on the left – hemiazygous vein, and in azygous aortic groove, *sulcus azygoaortalis* – thoracic duct, *ductus thoracicus.* Parietal layers of mediastinal pleura with lungs behind them are attached to the heart from both sides. There are large vessels at the top of the heart. In the anterior part the thymus gland (*glandula thymus*) is also attached to the heart, and adults have just the remains of it. Inferiorly, the heart is placed on the anterior folio (*folium anterius diaphragmaticum*) of the central tendon of the diaphragm. The system of coronary arteries and heart venous vessels form the third cardial circulation.

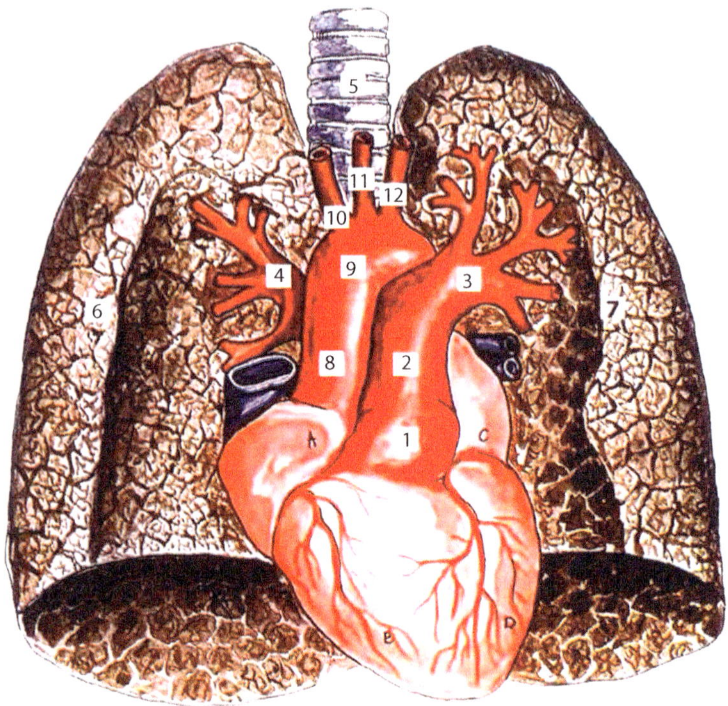

Figure 24 Heart and lungs.
1 – conus arterius; 2 – truncus pulmonalis; 3 – a. pulmonalis sinistra; 4 – a. pulmonalis dextra; 5 – trachea; 6 – pulmo dextrum; 7 – pulmo sinistrum; 8 – pars ascendens aortae; 9 – arcus aortae; 10 – truncus brachiocephalicus; 11 – a. caroticus communis; 12 – a. subclavia

Congenital deformities of atrial septum and ventricles of the heart. The size of hiatuses varies from several mm to 2 cm and more. They may be closed with functioning valves having *chorda tendinea* and its special papillary muscle. In the absence of the interatrial and interventricular septum both atrioventricular hiatuses merge into one. The artrial septal defect with stenotic mitral valve is characterized by hypoplasia of the left ventricle. In such cases, there is a blood excess in the right heart and pulmonary circuit.

Ascending aorta. *Aorta ascendens* starts from the left ventricle at the level of the third intercostal space. It is placed behind the breast bone. It is 5–6 cm long. It turns left and back, passing into the aortic arch (*arcus aortae*) at the level of the second right sternocostal joint. The ascending

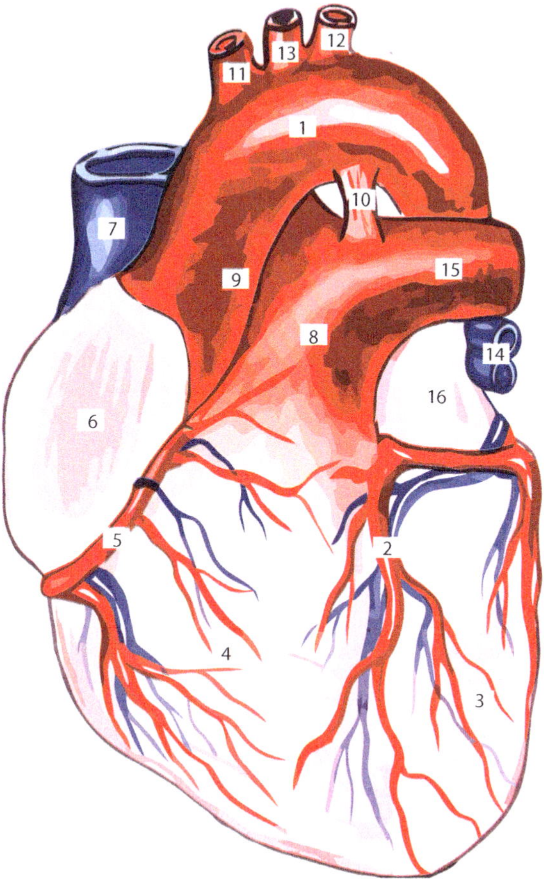

Figure 25 Heart.
1 – arcus aortae; 2 – a. coronaria dextra; 3. ventriculus sinister; 4 – ventriculus dexter; 5 - a. coronaria dextra; 6 – auricular dextra; 7 – v. cava superior; 8 – truncus pulmonalis; 9 – a. asscendens; 10 – lig. arteriale; 11 – truncus brachiocephalicus; 12 – a. subclavia sinistra; 13 – a. carotis communis sinistra; 14 – vv. pulmonalis sinister; 16 – auricular sinistra

aorta is the first but one out of three great vessels of the cardiac base: there is *v. cava superior* on the right and *a. pulmonalis* on the left.

Aortic arch. The aortic arch starts at the level of the second right sternocostal joint and forms an arch, the upper part of which corresponds to the center of the manubrium of sternum. The left innominate vein (*v. anonyma sinistra*) is attached to the arch superiorly; the transverse coronary sinus (*sinus transverses pericardii*), bifurcation of pulmonary

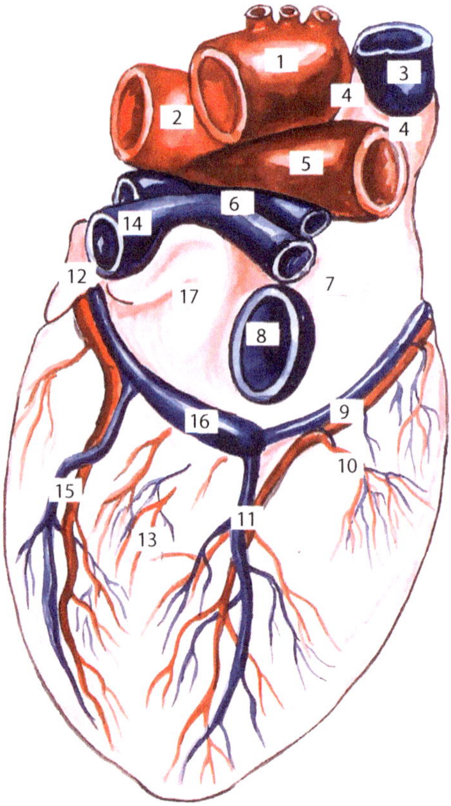

Figure 26 Heart. Back view.
1 – arcus aortae; 2 – a. pulmonalis sinistra; 3 – v. cava superior; 4 – переходная линия перикарда; 5 – a. pulmonalis dextra; 6 – vv. pulmonales dextrae; 7 – ventriculus dexter; 8 – v. cava inferior; 9 – a. coronaria dextra; 10 – vases ventriculi dextrae; 11 – средняя вена сердца и нисходящая ветвь правой венечной артерии; 12 – auricular sinistra; 13 – ventriculus sinister; 14 – vv. pulmonales sinistrae; 15 – vases ventriculi sinistrae; 16 – sinus coronary; 17 – atrium sinistrum

artery, left recurrent nerve (*n. recurrens sinister*), and obliterated Botallo duct (*ductus arteriosus (Botalli)*) pass inferiorly.

Aortic coarctation. Stenosis of aortic isthmus has different variations. In children stenosis may occur throughout several centimeters, in adults it comes to millimeters, while both *aa. subclaviae* are significantly enlarged to the size of the aorta. Then all branches of *aa. subclaviae* enlarge in diameter, particularly *truncus thyreocervicalis*, *truncus costocervicalis*, *a. transversa colli*, *a. thoracica*

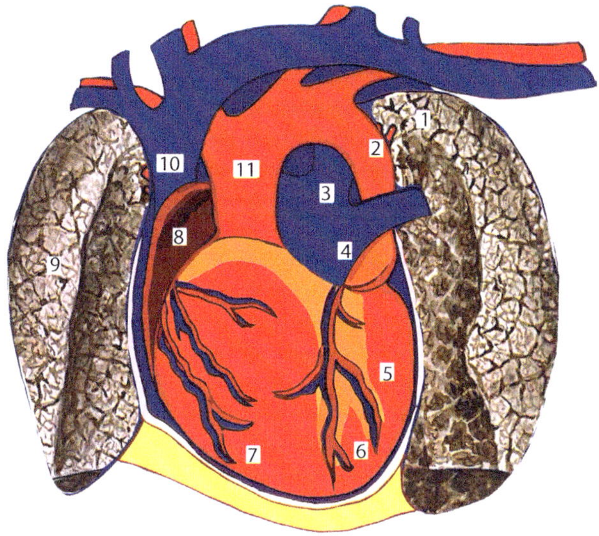

Figure 27 Syntopia of heart, big vessels and lungs.
1 – apex pulmonis sinistri; 2 – pars descendens aortae; 3 – ductus arteriosus; 4 – truncus pulmonalis; 5 – auricular sinistra; 6 – ventriculus; 8 – atrium dextrum; 9 – pulmo dexter; 10 – v. cava superior; 11 – pars ascendens aortae

interna – abdominal wall branches. All intercostal and lumbal arteries, as well as neurocanal and spinal cord vessels, are significantly expanded.

Arterial duct. *Ductus arteriosus (Botalli)* or Botallo duct is the anastomosis between the aortic arch and pulmonary artery, which has great importance in the uterine circulation. In a child of 3–6 months it is desolated and transforms into obliterated arterial ligament (*lig. arteriosum*).

In case of patent ductus arteriousus, some part of the blood from the aorta is flushed into pulmonary artery. As a result, systemic circuit is undersupplied with blood, while pulmonary circuit receives an excessive amount of it.

Main pulmonary artery, *A. Pulmonalis,* starts from right ventricle pulmonary cone (*conus arteriosus*). It lies on the left of the ascending aorta. Its origin corresponds to the second intercostal space on the left.

Pulmonary artery stenosis. In case of such a defect, there is hypertension in the right ventricle, which causes myocardial hypotrophy, the time of blood ejection into the pulmonary artery is increased and the whole cycle is broken.

Fallot's tetralogy. Congenital heart disease, consisting of a part of right ventricle obstruction, ventricular septal defect, aortic dextraposition, and right ventricular hypertrophy. In this case, dark blood from venae cavae mainly runs into the aorta through this defect. Aerated blood is mixed with dark blood, which leads to cyanosis, dyspnea and many other symptoms, common for this defect.

Superior vena cava. *V. cava superior* is formed by the junction of two brachiocephalic veins (*vv. brachiocephalicae dextra et sinistra*) at the level of the first costal cartilage attachment to the breast bone. It is 4-5 cm long. A big number of its valves can be found at the junction of the subclavian and internal jugular veins. It runs into the right atrium at the level of the third costal cartilage. Its inferior part enters into the pericardial cavity lower than the level of *v. azygos* entrance.

Inferior vena cava. The inferior vena cava (*v. cava inferior*) perforates the diaphragm passing through the inferior vena cava foramen or quadrangular foramen (*foramen venae cavae inferioris s. quadrilaterum*) and enters the pericardial cavity. Then above, it runs into the inferior part of the right atrium.

Phrenic nerves. The phrenic nerve (*n.phrenicus*) goes off the cervical plexus, along the anterior surface of the anterior scalene muscle, goes down and penetrates the thoracic cavity through the superior thoracic foramen.

The right phrenic nerve, lying alongside *a. pericardiacophrenica*, passes between the right mediastinal pleura and the superior vena cava.

The left phrenic nerve, also getting along with *a. pericardiacophrenica*, penetrates the thoracic cavity at the front of the aortic arch and lies between the left mediastinal pleura and the pericard.

Trachea and bronchi. (Figures 28, 29). The trachea is spaced for 3–4 cm from the thoracic wall in the breast bone notch area, and for 6–12 cm in the area of bifurcation. It is divided into right and left main bronchi behind the aortic arch, forming trachea bifurcation, which is projected to the 4th–5th thoracic vertebrae (this level divides superior mediastinum and three inferior ones).

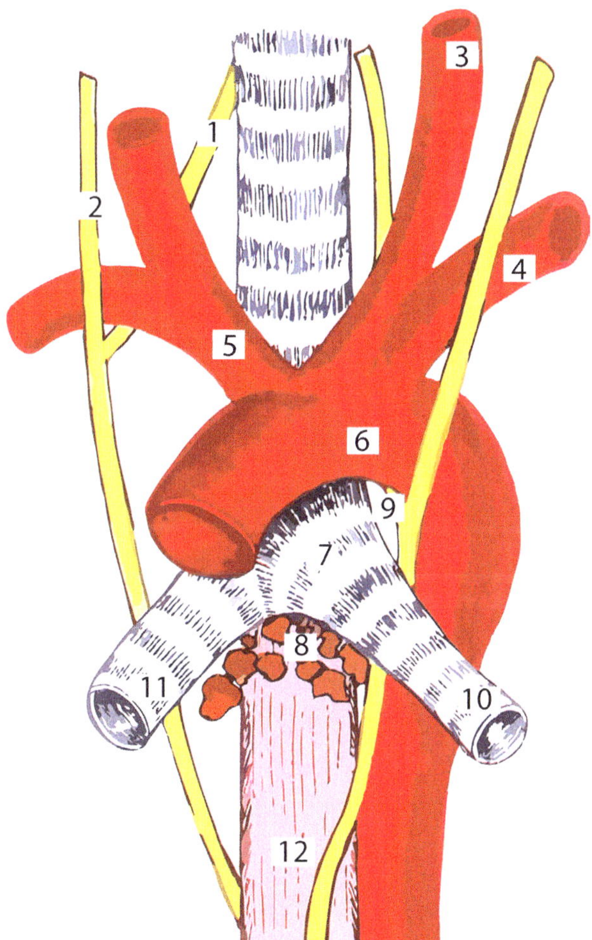

Figure 28 The relationship of the trachea, esophagus and aorta.
1 – n. recurrens dexter; 2 – n. vagus; 3 – a. carotis communis; 4 – a. subclavia; 5 – truncus brachiocephalicus; 6 – arcus aortae; 7 – bifurcation tracheae; 8 – nodi lymphatici tracheobronchiales; 9 – n. recurrens sinister; 10 – bronchus sinister; 11 – bronchus dexter; 12 – oesaphagus

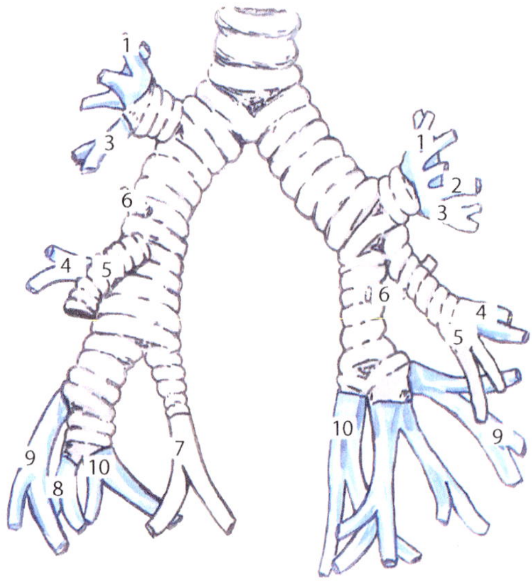

Figure 29 Pattern of segmental division of the bronchial tree.
1 – seg. apicale; 2 – seg. posterius; 3 – seg. anterius; 4 – seg. laterale (справа), lingulare superius (слева); 5 – seg. mediale; 6 – seg. apicale (superius); 7 – seg. basale mediale (cardiacum); 8 – seg. basale anterius; 9 – seg. basale laterale; 10 – seg. basale posterius

The right bronchus is shorter and wider than the left one; its direction almost coincides with the direction of the trachea. The right pulmonary artery passes in front of bifurcation, right atrium is placed downwards. *V. azygos* passes behind the posterior and superior walls of the right main bronchus. N. *vagus dexter* is placed along the right surface of trachea in the peritracheal tissue.

The aortic arch passes in front of the left bronchus, rounding it anteroposteriorly. Behind the left bronchus there is the esophagus, aortic arch and *n. vagus sinister*. Anteriorly, both bronchi are adjoined with the corresponding pulmonary artery.

Posterior mediastinum (Figures 30, 31). The anterior border of the posterior mediastinum is a pericard and trachea, the posterior border is a spinal column. Inside the mediastinum there is a thoracic aorta, azygos and hemiazygos veins, thoracic duct, esophagus, vagus nerves and sympathetic trunks with branching splanchnic nerves.

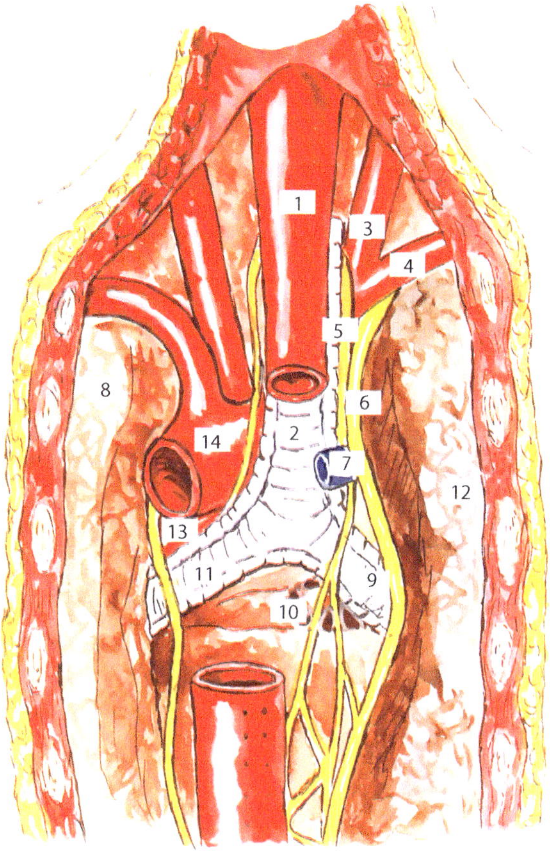

Figure 30 Posterior mediastinum.
1 – oesaphagus; 2 – trachea; 3 – a. carotis communis; 4 – a. subclavia; 5 – n. recurrens; 6 – n. vagus; 7 – v. azygos; 8 – pulmo sister; 9 – bronchus dexter; 10 – nodi lymphatici tracheobronchiales; 11 – bronchus sinister; 12 – pulmo dexter; 13 – a. pulmonalis sinistra; 14 – arcus aortae

Esophagus, *oesophagus*, extends from the 6th cervical vertebra to the 11th thoracic vertebra.

It presents a muscular tube with internal circular and external longitudinal muscle layers. The distance between teeth and esophagus beginning is approximately 15 cm. The length of esophagus in thoracic section is approximately 20 cm, while 3–4 cm is taken by the cervical section and 1–1.5 cm at abdominal one.

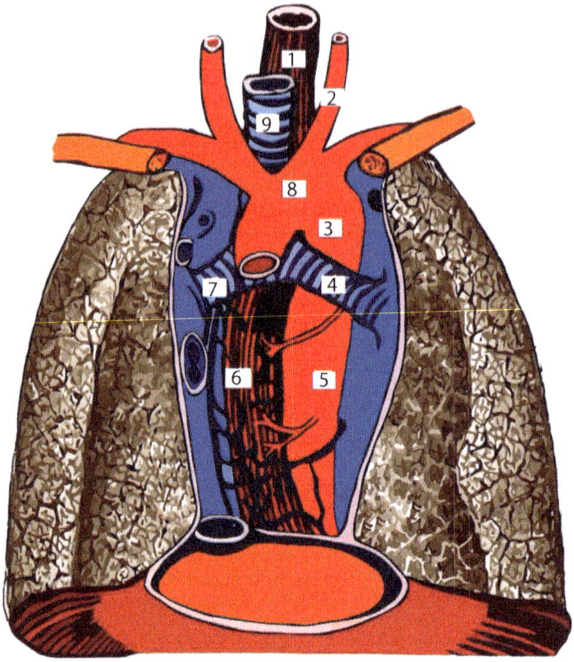

Figure 31 Blood supply of the middle and lower parts of the chest cavity.
1 – esophagus (pars cervicalis); 2 – a. carotis communis; 3 – pars descendens aortae (pars cervicalis); 4 – bronchus principalis sinister; 5 – rr. esophagales aortae; 6 – esophagus; 7 – bronchus principalis dexter; 8 – arcus aortae; 9 - trachea

Syntopy of esophagus. At the point where esophagus passes from neck to thoracic cavity the trachea is placed in front of the esophagus. In the posterior mediastinum esophagus starts gradual deviation on the left and at the level of the 5th thoracic vertebra it intersects the left bronchus, which is placed at its front. From this level, the thoracic aorta gradually passes onto the posterior surface of esophagus. On the top, up to the 4th thoracic vertebra, the esophagus is placed between the spinal column and trachea, which is adjacent anteriorly.

Below this level, the esophagus covers the notch between the azygos vein and aorta (*sulcus azygoaortalis*). The thoracic duct and spine are attached to the esophagus posteriorly; anteriorly it is covered by heart and vessels; on the right —*v. azygos*; on the left — thoracic part of aorta.

Esophageal atresia (Figure 32) is a developmental disease, when the upper segment of the esophagus is blind ended. Its lower segment more often communicates to the trachea. Anatomic shapes of esophageal atresia occur either without trachea communication or with thracheoesophageal fistula. With the latter option, the upper segment of the esophagus is placed at the level of the 2nd–3rd thoracic vertebra, and its lower segment is connected to the posterior or lateral trachea or bronchus wall by the fistulous tract.

Esophageal fistula. It is necessary to distinguish fistulas with respiratory organs, mediastinum, pleura and external fistulas. External fistulas in cervical section communicate with the esophagus, in the thoracic section – through pleural cavity. Fistulas may be of cancerous, traumatic, infective, and postsurgical origin.

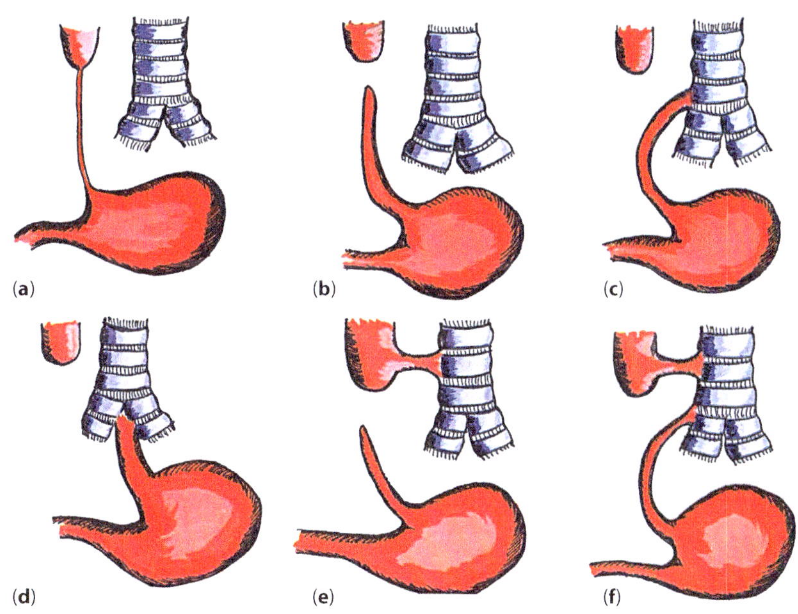

Figure 32 Types of esophagus atresia.
(a) aplasia of the esophagus; (b) the esophagus forms two isolated blind sacs; (c) the upper segment of the esophagus ends blindly, the lower segment is connected to the trachea (above the bifurcation) by the fistulous course; (d) the upper segment terminates blindly, the lower segment is connected to the bifurcation of the trachea by the fistulous course; (e) the upper segment is connected to the trachea, the lower is blind; (f) both segments of the esophagus are connected to the trachea by a fistulous course.

Descending aorta, *aorta descendens* is a third segment of aorta. It is subdivided into thoracic and abdominal. The thoracic aorta (*aorta thoracalis*) continues from the 4th to the 12th thoracic vertebrae. At the level of the 12th thoracic vertebra, the aorta passes into retroperitoneal space through aortic hiatus (*hiatus aorticus*). The thoracic aorta borders with the thoracic duct and azygos vein on the right, the hemiazygos vein on the left, the pericard and left bronchus anteriorly and thespinal column posteriorly. There are branches coming off the thoracic aorta to the thoracic organs – splanchnic branches (*rami visceralis*), and parietal branches (*rami parietals*). 9–10 pairs of intercostal arteries (*aa. intercostales)* belong to parietal branches.

The splanchnic branches are:

1. *Rami bronchiales* – bronchial branches, in a number of 2-4, most often 3 that supply bronchi and lungs with blood.
2. *Rami oesophageae* – esophageal arteries, in a number of 4-7, that supply esophageal wall with blood
3. *Rami pericardiaci* – pericard branches supply its posterior wall with blood.
4. *Rami mediastinales* – mediastinal branches that supply lymph gland and posterior mediastinum tissue with blood.

Azygos vein (*v. azygos*) is a direct continuation of the right ascending lumbar vein (*v. lumbalis ascendens dextra*). It goes up and is placed on the right of aorta, the thoracic duct and vertebral bodies, after passing between the internal and medial cruses of the diaphragm into the posterior mediastinum. On its way it accepts 9 inferior intercostal veins of the right side, as well as esophageal veins (*vv. oesophagea),* posterior bronchial veins (*vv. bronchiale posteriors*), and posterior mediastinum veins (*vv. mediastinales posteriors*). After rounding the right root of the lung back to front, the azygos vein opens into the superior vena cava (*v. cava superior*) at the level of the 4th-5th thoracic vertebrae. It may join the right atrium, right subclavian vein, right innominate vein, left innominate vein or left superior vena cava in case of *sinus inversus.*

Hemiazygos vein (*v. hemiazygos*) is a continuation of the left ascending lumbar vein (*v. lumbalis ascendens sinistra*), it penetrates through a tunnel between internal and medial cruses of the diaphragm and heads to posterior mediastinum. It goes behind the thoracic aorta, then up along the left side of the vertebral bodies and accepts the majority of intercostal veins from the left side.

The upper half of intercostal veins opens into the accessory vein (*v. hemiazygos accessoria*), which inflows directly into the azygos vein. Intersection with the spine hemiazigos vein is performed with different options: at the level of 8th, 9th, 10th or 11th thoracic vertebra.

Thoracic duct flow. The thoracic part of the thoracic duct (*pars thoracalis ductus thoracici*), which goes from the aortic hiatus to the thoracic inlet, is placed within the limits of posterior mediastinum. Then the thoracic duct lies in the azygoaortal notch (*sulcus azygoaortalis*). The thoracic duct is covered by the aorta edge near the diaphragm, anteriorly upwards it is covered with the posterior surface of the esophagus. In the thoracic section, it accepts left and right intercostal lymphatic vessels, collecting lymph from the breast posterior part, as well as the bronchomediastinal trunk (*truncus bronchomediastinalis*) running the lymph off the organs of the left part of the thoracic cavity. At the level of the 3rd, 4th, 5th thoracic vertebra the duct turns left to the left subclavian vein behind the esophagus, aortic arch and proceeds to the 7th cervical vertebra through *apertura thoracis superior.* The thoracic duct is usually 35-45 cm long of 0.5–1.7 cm in diameter. The thinnest part of the thoracic duct is in its middle, at the level of 4th–6th thoracic vertebra. One can find the thoracic duct in a form of a single trunk – monotrunk, paired thoracic duct – bitrunk, bifurcating one or glomerular thoracic ducts, forming one or several loops on its way. Single, double and triple loops and in rare cases even four loops can be found. The thoracic duct blood supply is performed by branches of intercostal arteries and esophagus arteries.

Vagus nerves. The left vagus nerve penetrates the thoracic cavity through the space between the common carotid artery and left subclavian artery and passes in front of the aortic arch. At the level of the inferior margin of the aorta, left *n. vagus* springs the left recurrent nerve (*n.recurrens sinister*), which passes around the aortic arch on the back and returns to the neck region. Then the left vagus nerve goes along the posterior surface of the left bronchus and the anterior surface of the esophagus.

The right vagus nerve enters the thoracic cavity, placing itself in the space between the right subclavian vessels – artery and vein. After passing around the subclavian artery in front, the vagus nerve springs *n. recurrens dexter,* which also returns to the neck at the back of the right subclavian artery. Below, the right vagus nerve passes behind the right bronchus and then lies onto the esophagus posterior surface.

The vagus nerves form loops on the esophagus and their strong and tense branches got the name of esophageal strings (*chordae oesophageae*).

The thoracic part of vagus nerve springs the following branches:

1. *Rami bronchiales anteriores* – anterior bronchial branches that head along anterior surface of bronchus to lung and form anterior pulmonary plexus (*plexus pulmonalis anterior*) together with branches of sympathetic trunk.

2. *Rami bronchiales posteriores* – posterior bronchial branches that also inosculate with branches of sympathetic trunk and enter lung hilum, where they form posterior pulmonary plexus (*plexus pulmonalis posterior*).

3. *Rami oesophagei* – esophageal branches that form anterior esophageal plexus (*plexus oesophageus anterior),* at the anterior surface of the esophagus (by the left vagus nerve). Similar plexus —*plexus oesophageus posterior* (by the right vagus nerve) is placed at the posterior surface of esophagus.

4. *Rami pericardiaci* – pericardium branches are sent in the form of small branches and innervate the heart sac.

Sympathetic trunks *Truncus sympathicus* – paired formation is placed alongside of the spinal column. Out of all organs of the posterior mediastinum, it is placed most laterally and corresponds to the heads of ribs level.

Each ganglion of sympathetic trunk (*ganglion trunci sympathicis. vertebrale)* sends white communicating branch (*ramus communicans albus*) and grey communicating branch (*ramuscommunicansgriseus*). The white communicating branch is presented by medullated fibres, passing through ventral root (*radix anterior*) to cells of *ganglion vertebrale.* These fibres are called preganglionic fibres (*fibrae preganglionares).* Grey communicating branch (*ramus communicans griseus)* carries nonmedullated fibres from *ganglion vertebrale* and heads as a part of the spinal nerve. These fibers are called postganglionic fibers (*fibrae postganglionares*).

Splanchnic nerves (Figure 33):

1. *N. splanchnicus major* – the greater splanchnic nerve starts with five roots from the 5th to the 9th thoracic ganglion. After inosculation into one trunk, the nerve heads to the diaphragm and penetrates the abdominal cavity between *crus mediale* and *crus intermedium diaphragmatis* and takes part in celiac plexus (*plexus solaris*) formation.

2. *N. splanchnicus minor* – the lesser splanchnic nerve starts from the 10th to the 11th thoracic sympathetic ganglions and together with *n. splanchnicus major* penetrates the abdominal cavity, where it is partly included in *plexus solaris,* but mainly forms renal plexus (*plexus renalis*).

3. *N. splanchnicus imus, s. minimus, s. tertius* – an unpaired, small or third splanchnic nerve starts from the 12th thoracic sympathetic ganglion and also enters *plexus renalis.*

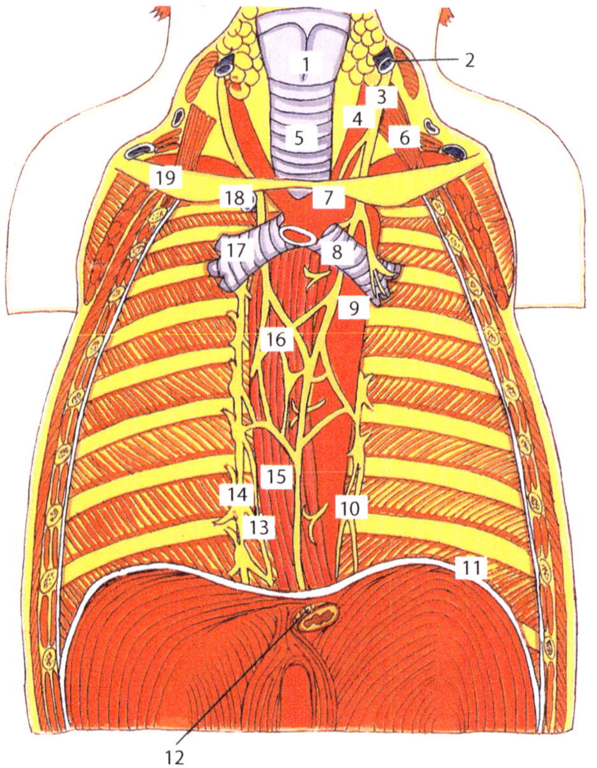

Figure 33 Topography of the organs of the posterior mediastinum. Front view.
1 – larynx; 2 – v. jugularis interna; 3 – n. vagus; 4 – a. carotis communis; 5 – trachea; 6 – m. scalenus anterior; 7 – arcus aortae; 8 – bronchus principalis sinister; 9 – pars descendens aortae (pars rhotacica); 10 – truncus vagakis anterior; 13 – n. splanchnicus major; 14 – truncus sympathicus; 15 – esophagus; 16 – plexus esophagealis; 17 – bronchus principalis dexter; 18 – v. azygos; 19 – clavicula

Specific features of posterior mediastinum organs in children. The heart of a newborn is round in shape; due to the high position of the diaphragm the heart is placed horizontally, later it takes an oblique position. The trachea is relatively wide, supported by open-ended cartilaginous rings and wide muscular membrane.

Children's bronchi are narrow, the angle of junction between bronchi and trachea is the same, and so the extraneous bodies may get into either left or right bronchus. Then, the angle changes, and the extraneous bodies can be found in the right bronchus more often, as it is a trachea continuation. A newborn's esophagus starts at the level of cartilage between the 3rd and 4th cervical vertebrae. At the age of 2, the superior margin is at the level of the 4th–5th vertebra, and by 12 years it is at the level of the 6th–7th cervical vertebrae, as in adults.

The esophagus has an irregular cylindrical shape. A newborn's thymus is 12 gr and grows up to puberty. Superiorly, it is projected 1–1.5 cm above the manubrium of sternum; inferiorly, it reaches the 3rd, 4th, or 5th rib.

Mediastinal cellular spaces. The anterior mediastinum cellular tissue surrounds the trachea and bronchi, forming the peritracheal space, which inferior margin is formed by fascial compartment of the aortic arch and root of the lung. It contains blood vessels, lymphatic glands, branches of vagus and sympathetic nerves and extraorgan nervous plexus.

There is periesophageal cellular space in the posterior mediastinum. Anteriorly, it is limited by preoesophageal fascia, posteriorly – by retroesophageal one, laterally – by mediastinal ones. Fascial spurs containing blood vessels go from the esophagus to fascial bed walls. The periesophageal space is a continuation of retrovisceral neck cellular tissue and is focalized in the upper section between the esophagus and spinal column, and in lower section between descending aorta and esophagus. Herewith, the cellular tissue does not go beneath the 9th–10th thoracic vertebrae.

Parietal lymph nodes (Figure 34). Parietal nodes are placed at the posterior wall of the thoracic cage – prevertebral (*nodi lymphatici prevertebrales*), and intercostal (*nodi lymphatici intercostales*); at the anterior wall – paramammary ones (*nodi lymphatici paramammarii*); and parasternal ones (*nodi lymphatici parasternalis*); at the inferior wall – superior phrenic lymph nodes (*nodi lymphatici phrenici superiors*).

Visceral nodes. There are prepericardial and lateral pericardial nodes (*nodi lymphatici prepericardiales et pericardiales laterals*), anterior mediastinal nodes (*nodi lymphatici mediastinails anteriores*), and posterior mediastinal nodes (*nodi lymphatici mediastinals posteriors*).

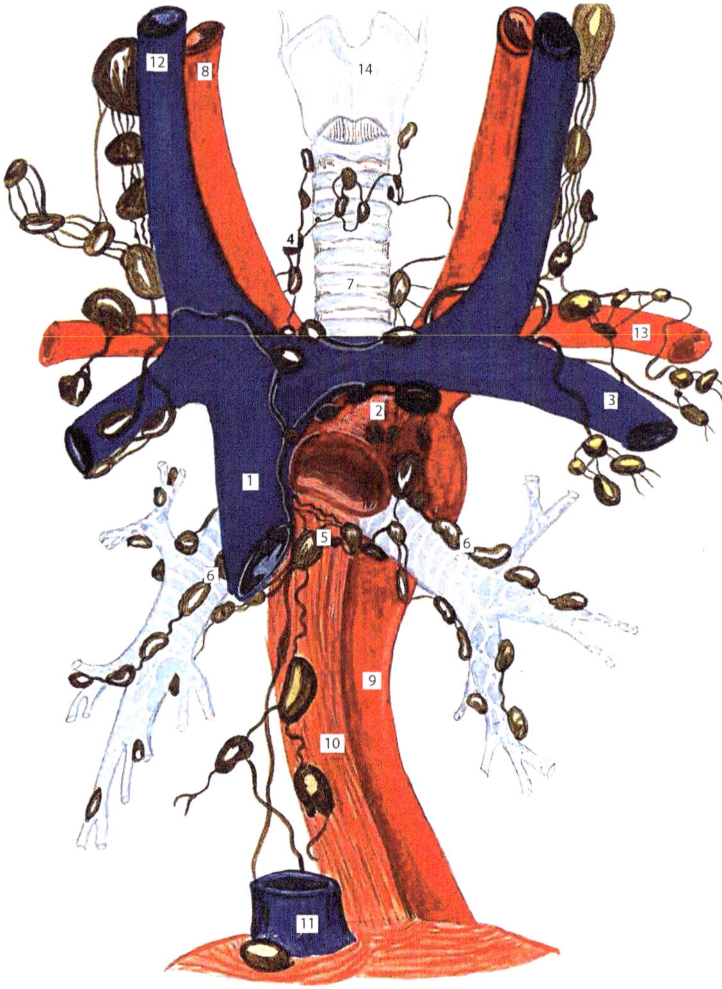

Figure 34 Organs and lymph nodes of the mediastinum.
1 – v. cava superior; 2 – arcus aortae; 3 – v. subclavia; 4 – nodi lymphatici bifurcations; 6 – nodi lymphatici bronchiales; 7 – trachea; 8 – a. carotis communis; 9 – pars aortae descendens; 10 – oesophagus; 11 – v. cava inferior; 12 – v. jugularis interna; 13 – a. subclavia; 14 – cartilage thyroidea

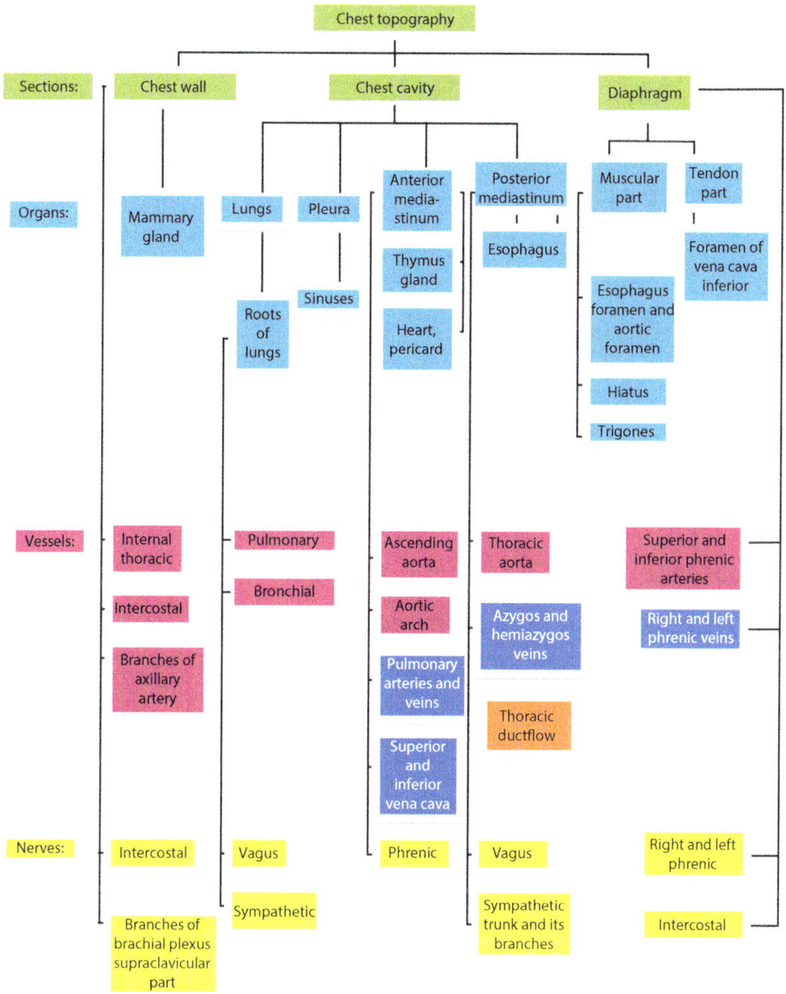
Chest topography
Sections:
Chest wall
Chest cavity
Diaphragm
Organs:
Mammary gland
Lungs
Pleura
Anterior media-stinum
Posterior mediastinum
Muscular part
Tendon part
Thymus gland
Esophagus
Foramen of vena cava inferior
Sinuses
Roots of lungs
Heart, pericard
Esophagus foramen and aortic foramen
Hiatus
Trigones
Vessels:
Internal thoracic
Pulmonary
Ascending aorta
Thoracic aorta
Superior and inferior phrenic arteries
Bronchial
Intercostal
Aortic arch
Azygos and hemiazygos veins
Right and left phrenic veins
Branches of axillary artery
Pulmonary arteries and veins
Thoracic ductflow
Superior and inferior vena cava
Nerves:
Intercostal
Vagus
Phrenic
Vagus
Right and left phrenic
Sympathetic
Sympathetic trunk and its branches
Intercostal
Branches of brachial plexus supraclavicular part

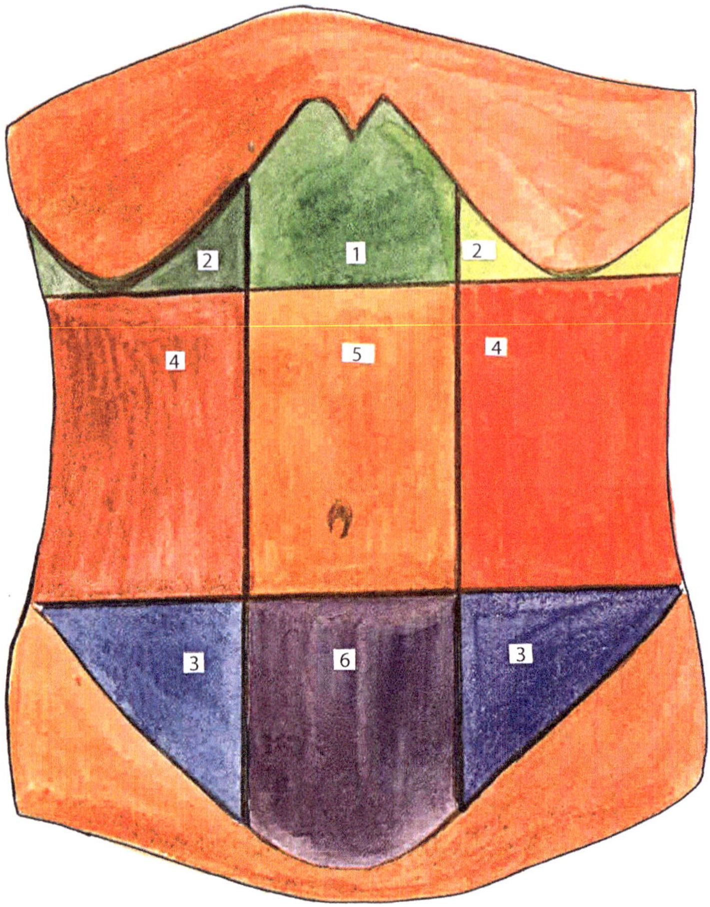

Figure 35 Sections of anterior lateral abdomen wall.
1 – reg. epigastrica; 2 – reg. hypochondrica; 3 – regio inguinalis; 4 – reg. abdominalis; 5 – reg. umbilicalis; 6 – reg. pubica.

small intestine loops, and lower pole of right kidney are projected to *regio lumbalis dextra*.

The bladder (filled up), lower ureter, uterus, small intestine loops are projected to *regio suprapubica*. The blind gut, subileum, vermicular appendix, and right *ureter are projected to regio inguinalis dextra*. The sigmoid colon, small intestine loops, and left ureter are projected to *regio inguinalis sinistra*.

Layers of regions and their characteristics. Sectional (layer by layer) topography within the bounds of rectus abdominis muscle. (Figure 36):

1. **Above semicircular line**: *1) derma, 2) panniculus adiposus; 3) fascia superficialis; 4) fascia propria m. oblique*

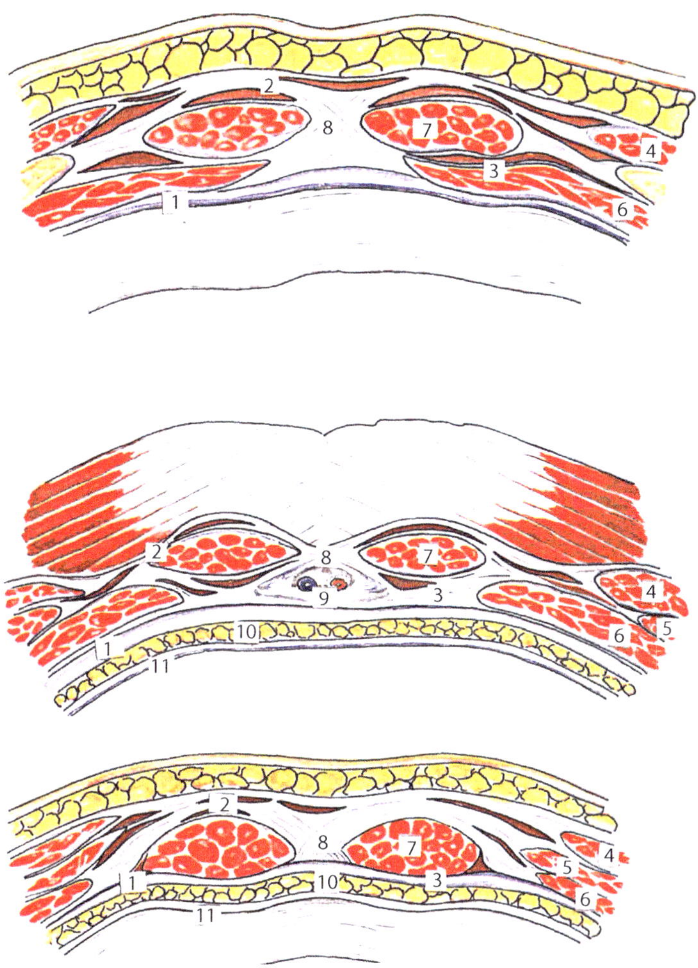

Figure 36 Transversal sections of anterior abdominal wall at different levels.
1 – fascia transversa; 2 – lamina anterior vag. m. recti abdominis; 3 – lamina posterior vag. m. recti abdominis; 4 – m. obliquus externus abdominis; 5 – m. obliquus internus abdominis; 6 – m. transversus abdominis; 7 – m. rectus abdominis; 8 – linea alba; 9 – lig. teres hepatis; 10 – tela subserosa; 11 – peritoneum

abdominis externi; 5) paries anterior vaginae m. recti abdominis; 6) m. rectus abdominis; 7) paries posterior vaginae m. recti abdominis; 8) fascia transversa; 9) stratum adiposum praeperitonaeles; 10) peritoneum parietale;

2. **Below the semicircular line:** the layers are the same, but the anterior wall of rectus sheath is composed of three adherent aponeuroses of abdominal muscles; the posterior wall is missing.
3. **Ectad of rectus abdominis muscle**: *1) derma; 2) panniculus adiposus; 3) fascia superficialis; 4) fascia Thompsoni; 5) fascia propria obliqui abdominis externi; 6) m. obliquus abdominis externus; 7) stratum fasciale intermusculare; 8) m. obliquus abdominis internus; 9) stratum fasciale intermusculare; 10) m. transversus abdominis; 11) fascia transversa; 12) stratum adiposum praeperitonaeles; 13) peritoneum parietale;*
4. **Umbilicus area:** *1) derma; 2) fascia umbilicalis; 3) peritoneum parietale.*

Sectional topography of inguinal area (Figure 46): *1) derma; 2) panniculus adiposus; 3) fascia superficialis; 4) fascia Thompsoni; 5) fascia propria m. obliqui abdominis externi; 6) aponeurosus m.obliqui abdominis externi;* 7) inguinal canal itself; 8) with men — *funiculus spermaticus;* with women — *lig. teres uteri; 9) lig.inguinale; 10) m.obliquus internus abdominis et m. abdominis transversus; 11) fascia transversa; 12) stratum adiposum praeperitoneale; 13) peritoneum parietale.*

Topography of the inferior section of anterior abdominal wall is presented in Figure 38.

The skin is relatively thin, easily plicated, significantly mobile and flexible. The abdomen subdermal tissue (*tela subcutanea abdominis),* or subcutaneous fat, often contains a large quantity of fat. The exception is the median line, where the abdominal raphe is projected – there is usually less fat in it, and the umbilicus, containing no fat at

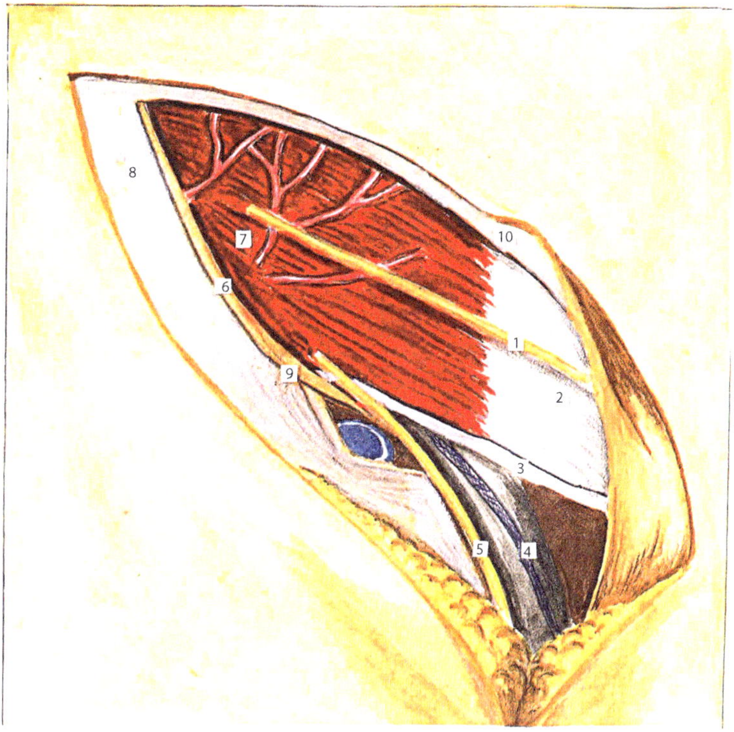

Figure 37 Topography of inguinal area.
1 – n. iliohypogastricus; 2 – aponeurosis m. obliquus externus abdominis; 3 – lig. reflexum; 4 – funiculus spermaticus; 5 – n. ilioinguinalis; 6 – lig. inguinalis; 7 – m. obliquus internus abdominis; 8 – aponeurosis m. obliquus externus abdominis; 9 – margo inferior m. obliquus externus abdominis; 10 – margo superior aponeurosis m. obliquus externus abdominis.

all. Subcutaneous fat layer is more developed in the lower half of the abdomen.

The superficial layer of tissue is of cellular structure, the deep one is of layered structure. Superficial fascia consists of two laminas: superficial and deep one. The superficial lamina is thin and loose; it spreads onto neighboring areas. The deep lamina is well marked in a lower part of the abdomen and is known as fascia. This lamina is often called Thompson fascia.

The deep lamina of fascia is attached to the inguinal ligament, and due to this inguinal hernias do not descend below the inguinal ligament. Superficial veins and nerves pass between layers of superficial fascia

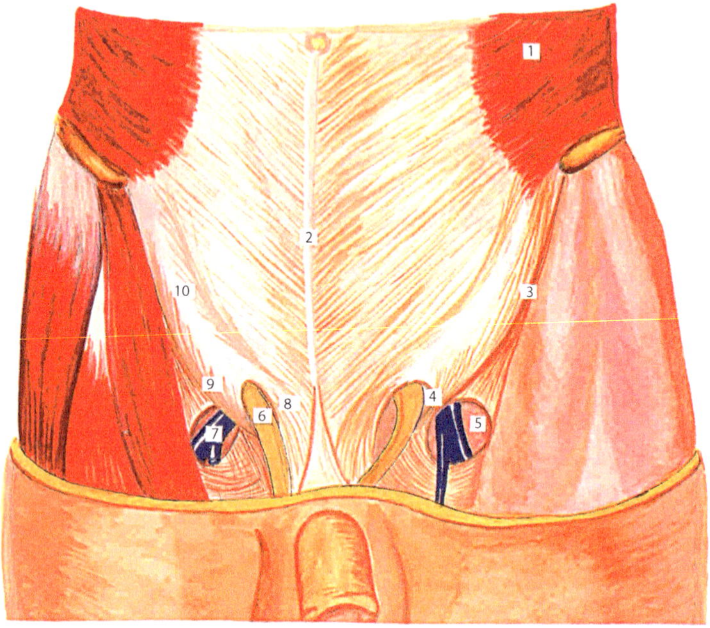

Figure 38 Topography of inferior section of anterior abdominal wall.
1- m. obliquus externus abdominis; 2 – linea alba; 3 – lig. inguinale; 4 – anullus inguinalis superficialis; 5 – foramen externus canalis femoralis; 6 – funiculus spermaticus; 7 – v. femoralis; 8 – margo superior (internus) aponeurosis m. obliquus externus abdominis; 9 – margo inferior (externus) aponeurosis m. obliquus externus abdominis; 10 – aponeurosis m. obliquus externus abdominis.

and inside subcutaneous fat. Inferiorly, the superficial epigastric artery (*a. epigastrica superficialis*) and superficial circumflex iliac artery (*a. circumflexa ilium superficialis*), branching off the femoral artery, begin from the hip anterior region to the abdomen inguinal region. The former heads to the umbilical region, the latter goes towards *spina iliaca anterior superior* and the skin of this region. Both arteries have to be transected in case of inguinal hernia operations.

Specific features of children. Compared to adults, a child's anterior wall is insufficiently formed and suffers significant age peculiarities during its development. Regardless of gender, the infant's abdomen has a form of inverted conoidal frustum. The abdominal wall is slightly bulging forward and hangs down because of insufficient development of muscles and aponeurosis. The bulge of the anterior abdominal wall will gradually disappear in the future due to age-specific muscular hyperstenia.

The skin of a child's abdominal wall is thin, subcutaneous fat is well developed, but is spread unevenly. Superficial fascia of the abdominal wall is very thin and has only one layer above the umbilicus. It consists of two layers below the umbilicus level. The abdominal fascia is thin and loose. It gradually thickens with age. The abdomen muscles are poorly developed and hard to differentiate.

Infants' abdominal raphe is relatively wide and of small thickness. The umbilical ring appears as a result of abdominal raphe formation by separation of aponeurotic fibers in this place, forming semi-oval or round defect of anterior abdominal wall.

A child's inguinal canal is relatively short, but wide.

Neurovascular fascicles. Skin innervation is performed by intercostal nerves (from the 7th to 12th) and branches of ilio-hypogastric nerve, *n. iliohypogastricus.*

Arterial and venous anastomosises (Figure 39). Superficial veins, accompanying the arteries, form numerous anastomosises in hypoderm. Most significantly, these veins inosculate with veins from other body regions – breast and lower limb. In particular, there are important anastomosises of *vv. thoracoepigastricae*, which start next to the umbilicus and flow into axillary vein or in *v. thoracica lateralis,* i.e., superior vena cava system, and of *vv. epigasricae superilciales*, flowing in femoral vein, i.e., inferior vena cava system. These are cavo-caval anastomosises, coming to operation in case of misperfusion (occlusion) of superior or inferior vena cava.

Anastomosises of anterior superficial veins of the abdominal wall with *vv. paraumbilicales*, starting from the umbilicus in round ligament of liver and flowing in porta (*v. portae)* are equally important. These veins form portocaval anastomosis.

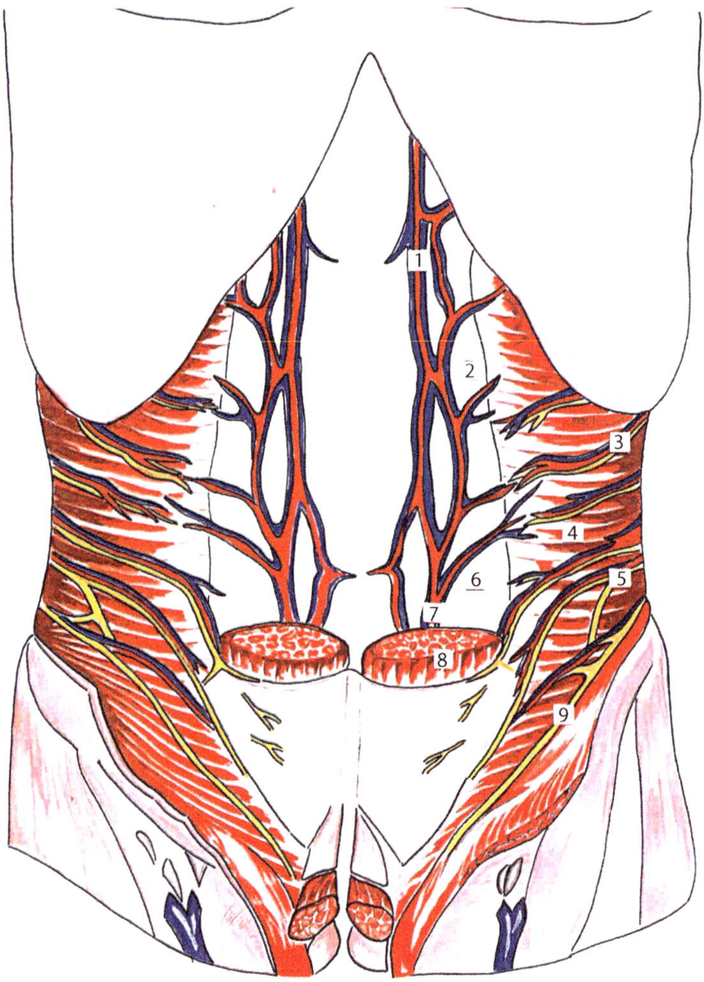

Figure 39 Anterior abdominal wall blood supply and anastomoses.
1 – a. et v. epigastrica superior; 2 – paries posterior vag. m. recti abdominis; 3 – aa., vv. Intercostales posteriors et nn. intercostales; 4 – m. transverses abdominis; 5 – n. iliohypogastricus; 6 – linea arcuata; 7 – a.et v. epigastrica superior; 8 – m. rectu sabdominis; 9 – n. ilioinguinalis; 10 – m. obliquus internus abdominis; 11 – aponeurosis obliqi interni abdominis; 12 – parieces anterior et posterior vag. m. recti abdomen

Inosculation of superficial veins with deep *vv. epigastricae superior et inferior* is also significant. The expansion of the anterior abdominal wall subcutaneous veins network is a result of blood drainage disturbance in vena cava or porta veins. In such cases, they protrude through the skin in a form of serpentine plexuses within the umbilical region (such plexuses are called "Medusa head").

Cellular spaces: rectus sheath (anterior and posterior fissures), hiatus between *m. obliquus internus et m. transverses abdominis,* retropubic and vesical spaces, layer of tissue between parietal peritoneum and *f. endoabdominalis.*

Peritoneal folds and fossas at internal surface of anterior lateral abdomen wall (Figures 40, 41). Round ligament of liver is a peritoneal

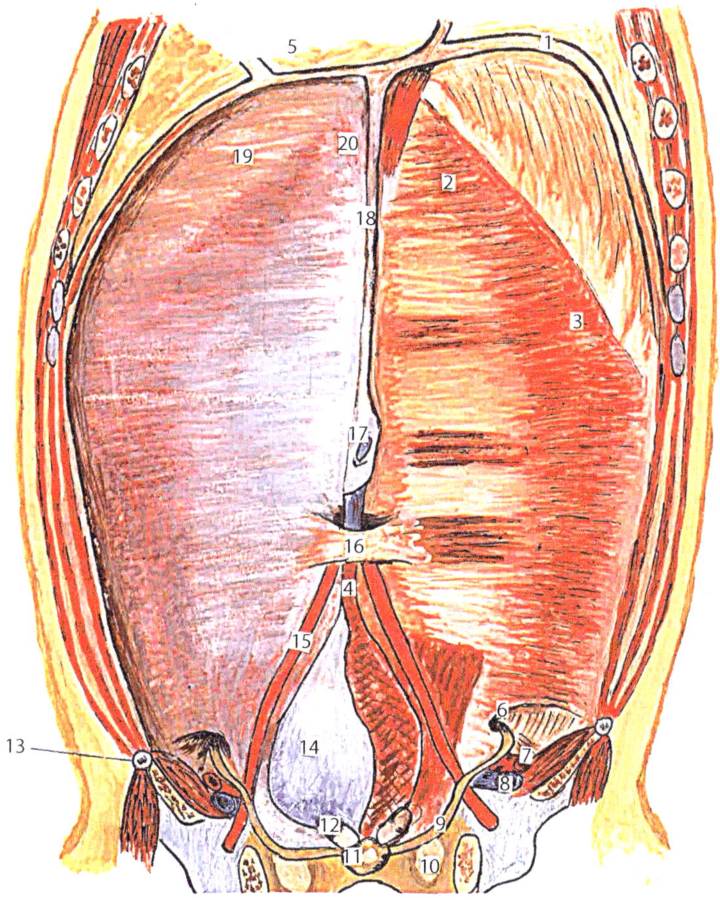

Figure 40 Internal surface of anterior abdominal wall. Removed peritoneum in the right half.
1.diaphragma; 2. vag. m. recti abdominis (lam. posterior); 3. m. transverses abdominis; 4. urachus; 5. a. umbilicalis; 6. annulus inguinalis profundus; 7. a. iliaca externa; 8. v. femoralis; 9. funiculus spermaticus; 10. foramen obturatorium; 11. prostata; 12. vesicula seminales; 13. spina iliaca anterior superior; 14. vesica urinaria; 15. plica umbilicalis; 16. fascia umbilicalis; 17. v. umbilicalis; 18. lig. fulciformis hepatic; 19. arcus costalis; 20.processus xiphoideus.

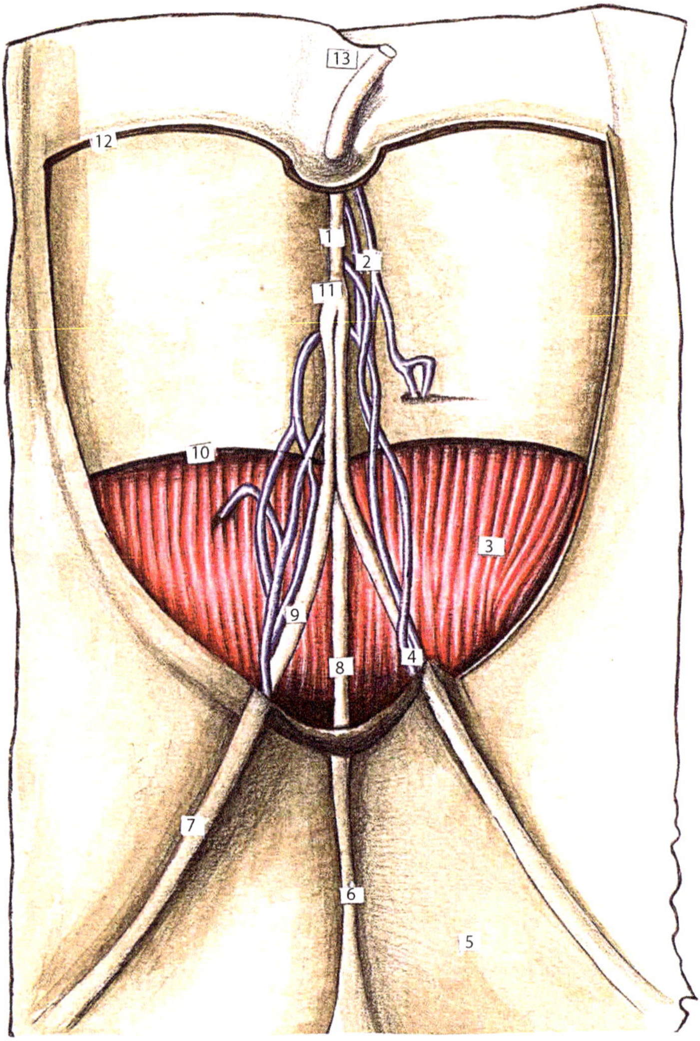

Figure 41 The topography of the anterolateral abdominal wall.
1 – vag. n. recti abdomini; 2 – m. rectus abdominis; 3 – intersection tendinis; 4 – m. obliquus internus abdominis; 5 – m. obliquus externus abdominis; 6 – m. pyramidalis; 7 – fascia transversa; 8 – linea semicircularis; 9 – linea semilunaris; 10 – n. transversus abdominis; 11 – linea alba abdominis; 12 – arcus costalis.

fold (*lig. teres hepatis*), going from the umbilicus in up and right direction, and then passing through umbilical fissure (*fissura lig. teretis hepatis*). It contains part of obliterated umbilical vein (*v. umbilicalis*) and is passed by *vv. paraumbilicales.*

Median umbilical fold ((*plica umbilicalis mediana*) is an unpaired peritoneal fold above closed urachus, going from the apex of the urinary bladder to the umbilicus. Medial umbilical fold (*plica umbilicalis medialis*) – is a fold above *a. umbilicalis,* obliterated throughout the major part of its length, except for a small section in a place where the artery origins from internal iliac artery. This fold goes from the lateral surface of the bladder to the umbilicus.

Lateral umbilical fold (*plica umbilicalis lateralis*) is a peritoneal fold above *a. et v. epigastricae inferiores*. There are peritoneal notches, or fossas, at internal surface of anterior abdominal wall between the above-mentioned peritoneal folds.

Supravesical fossa (*fossa supravesicalis*) is paired, placed above the bladder and bounded medially by *plica umbilicalis mediana* and laterally by *plica umbilicalis medialis*. Medial inguinal fossa (*fossa inguinalis medialis*) is paired, placed between *plica umbilicalis medialis* and *plica umbilicalis lateralis*. Medial inguinal fossa projectively corresponds to external inguinal ring, placed ectad of pubic spine. The lateral inguinal fossa (*fossa inguinalis lateralis*) is also paired, placed ectad of *plica umbilicalis lateralis*. It is attached to the deep inguinal ring and projected above the middle of the inguinal ligament.

Inguinal and umbilical canals and their special features in children. The inguinal canal is a fissure between the broad abdomen muscles above the medial half of the inguinal ligament. The inguinal canal has four walls: anterior, posterior, superior and inferior and two foramens: subcutaneous abdominal ring and peritoneal one.

The anterior wall is formed by aponeurosis of abdominal external oblique muscle, posterior one – by transverse fascia, superior one – by overhanging free borders of the abdominal internal oblique muscle and transverse abdominal muscle, inferior one – by canal of fallopian arch.

Subcutaneous abdominal ring (*annulus inguinalis subcutaneus*) is formed by two cruses of splitted aponeurosis of abdominal external oblique muscle: superior (*crus superius*) and inferior (*crus inferius*).

larger. Anatomic pre-condition of the formation of congenita inguinal hernia is nonclosure processus vaginalis of peritoneum. It is the prepared sack for inguinal hernia. Pre-condition of the formation of the strangulated inguinal hernia is a narrow gate of hernia. Pre-condition of the formation of postoperative hernia is inflammation of operating sutures, enhanceable physical activity after an operation, insufficient quantity of restoring forces and low immunity, obesity, strong cough, vomiting, constipations in postoperative period.

Surgical anatomy of umbilical hernias, direct and slanting inguinal and femoral hernias. The sack of hernia is situated in an inguinal channel among the elements of spermatic cord under inguinal hernia. The sack of hernia is situated inwardly from a spermatic cord under direct hernia. There are some signs to differentiate slanting and direct hernia: slanting hernia occurs at a young age more often, slanting hernia is one-sided usually, slanting hernia can go down in a scrotum at the protracted time of existence. Direct hernia occurs at an elderly age more often, direct hernia is bilateral usually, direct hernia cannot go down in a scrotum. Slanting hernia can be congenital. The sack of hernia is nonclosure processus vaginalis of peritoneum. A vascular lacuna is the basic place of formation of femoral hernia. More "weak" department of vascular lacuna is a femoral ring (anulus femoralis). A femoral ring is situated in the medial department of lacuna. It is delimited: medial - by a medial-lacunar copula, at the front - by an inguinal copula, behind - by a Cooper copula, lateral - by the vagina of femoral vein. A femoral ring is filled by fatty cellulose. The large lymph node of Rosenmuller-Pirogov is located in this area. The diameter of a femoral ring for women is 1.8 cm, for men is 1.2 cm.

Surgical Anatomy of Congenital Malformations of Anterior Lateral Abdominal Wall

Fistulas of umbilicus, hernia of umbilical cord. The fistulas of umbilicus are the congenital anomalies of the development. They are the result of nonclosure of vitelline canal or urinary canal. There are complete and incomplete fistulas. A complete umbilical fistula is complicated by the eversion of its mucous membrane. In scream and tension the wall of bowel opposite to the channel can fall out. This can result in a bowel obstruction. A part of the abdominal region organs is located in the shells of the umbilical cord under hernia of the umbilical cord. Sizes of the hernia sack can be from small (2–5 cm) to giant - 15–20 cm. A gate of hernia is an extended umbilical ring. The sizes of defect vary from a 1–2 cm to considerable. Hernia can be an elongated with a narrow gate, or semispherical depending on the sizes of defect of the umbilical ring. An umbilical cord passes to the apex of sack of hernia. There are three umbilical vessels in a sack before an abdominal region. Intestines, stomach, liver can be a content of hernia sack.

Abdominal Region Topography

Peritoneum and Abdominal Cavity Levels

An abdominal region is part of the abdominal cavity. This cavity is limited by the limits of the parietal leaf of the peritoneum. A peritoneum is a serosa. It covers the internal surface of the stomach walls and organs, which are located in the abdominal region. It forms the closed cavity. The peritoneal cavity has the character of the slot, which is usually filled by serofluid. The eritoneum consists of two sheets - parietal and visceral. Organs that are covered by the visceral peritoneum from every parties are located intraperitoneally. Organs which are covered by the visceral peritoneum from three parties are located mezoperitoneally. Organs which are covered by the visceral peritoneum from one side are located extraperitoneally. Organs which are located intraperitoneally and mezoperitoneally are organs of the abdominal region. Organs which occupy retroperitoneal position (it is a special case of extraperitoneal position), are organs of extraperitoneal space. It is traditionally opinion in a topographical anatomy.

Lig. Hepatoduodenale is a hepatoduodenal copula (Figure 42). It is one of three copulas of lesser omentum. This copula has a most

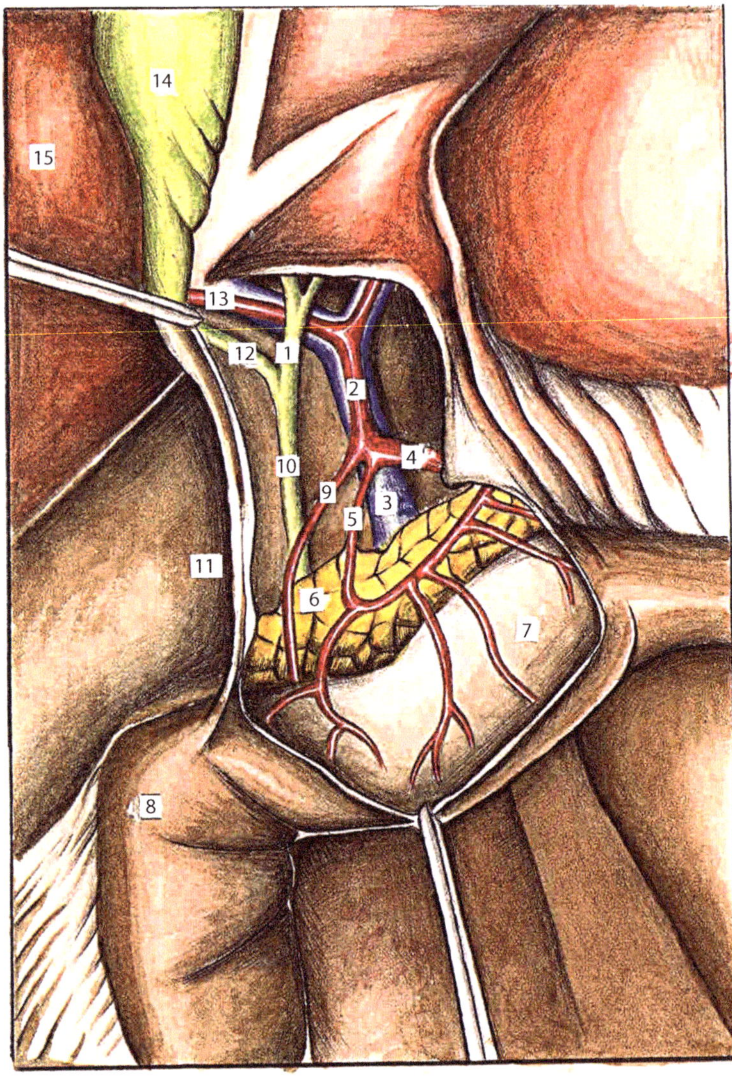

Figure 42 Content of hepatoduodenal copula.
1 – ductus hepaticus; 2 – a. hepatica propria; 3 – v. portae; 4 – a. hepatica communis; 5 – a. gastrica dextra; 6 – pancreas; 7 – gaster; 8 – duodenum; 9 – a. gastroduodenalis; 10 – ductus choledochus; 11 – ostium omentalis; 12 – ductus cysticus; 13 – r. a. hepatica propria dexter; 14 – vesica fellea; 15 – hepar.

meaning. Bilious channel (*ductus choledochus*), janitrix (*v. portae*) and own hepatic artery (*a. hepatica propria*) are located in this copula. Hepatoduodenal copula goes into to the hepatopyloric copula (*lig. hepatopyloricum*) on the left.

Lig. suspensorium duodeni is a suspensory copula of duodenum (**copula of Treytsa).** It goes from the left leg of lumbar department of the diaphragm to the duodenal-jejunal bend (*flexura duodenojejunalis*). A smooth muscle of the same name (*m. Duodenojejunalis*) lies in the interior of the suspensory copula of duodenum. This muscle is a muscle of supporting a duodenum.

Omentum majus **(epiploon)** are duplicatura of peritoneum, which descends from the large curvature of the stomach. It covers the loops of the thin bowel. This duplicatura accretes with a transverse colon. The cavity of epiploon has next borders. The front border is *lig. gastrocolicum*. The rear boundary is presented by the parietal peritoneum. The lower boundary is the transverse colon and its mesentery. The upper boundary is a gastro pancreatic copulas with a gastro pancreatic opening. This opening is located between copulas. The left boundary is a splenic eversion of the cavity of epiploon (*recessus lienalis cavi omenti majoris*). The right boundary is a pancreatic-duodenal pocket of the cavity of epiploon (recessus *pancreaticoduodenalis cavi omenti majoris*).

There are four eversions in the cavity of epiploon: 1) upper eversion is a gastropancreatic eversion (*recessus gastropancreaticus*); 2) bottom eversion (*recessus inferior*); 3) on the left is a splenic eversion (*recessus lienalis*) and gate of spleen; 4) on the right is a pancreatic-duodenal eversion (*recessus pancreaticoduodenalis*).

The epiploon is located in the left half of the stomach, along the lower edge of the transverse colon in children. It is short. It covers the loops of bowels only partly. Sizes of epiploon grow till 2–3 years. But sheets of peritoneum remained very thin. A fatty cellulose between them is almost absent.

Omentum minus (lesser omentum) - is a duplicatura of the peritoneum. It stretches from the gate of the liver. It stretches from the back half of the left sagittal furrow of the liver to the small curvature of stomach also. And it stretches to the initial department of horizontal part of the

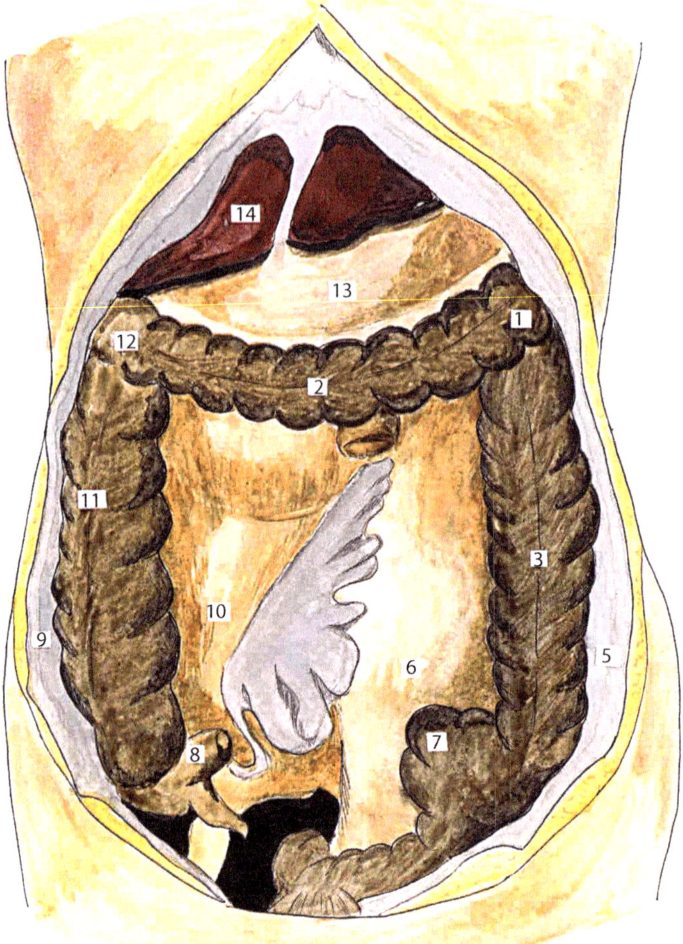

Figure 44 The ground floor of the abdominal cavity.
1 – flexura lienalis intestine crassi; 2 – colon transversum; 3 – colon descendens; 4 – mesenterium intestine tenue; 5 – canalis lateralis sinister; 6 – sinus mesenteries sinister; 7 – colon sigmoideun; 8 – caecum; 9 – canalis lateralis dexter; 10 – colon ascendens; 11 – flexura hepatis intestine crassi; 12 – ventriculus; 13 – hepar.

hepatis. Outside that bag is limited by a muscular part of diaphragm, *pars muscularis diaphragmatis*. This bag quite often serves as a receptacle for subphrenic abscesses.

Bursa hepatica sinistra (a left hepatic bag) is located between the left stake of liver and diaphragm. Its borders are at the front – the muscular part of the diaphragm, *pars muscularis diaphragmatis*, behind – the left coronal copula of liver, *lig. coronarium hepatls sinistrum*, from within – suspending or falcate copula of liver, *lig. suspensorium s. falciforme hepatis*, outside – the left three-cornered copula of liver, *lig. triangulare hepatis sinistrum.*

Bursa pregastrica (a pre-stomach bag) is situated between a stomach and left lobe of liver. More exact borders are at the front - a lower surface of the left lobe of liver, behind - a front of wall of stomach, from above - an lesser omentus and gate of liver.

The right and left mesenteric sines, *sinus mesentericus dexter and sinus mesentericus sinister* are located in the ground floor of the abdominal region. Both sines have a three-cornered form. The right sine is limited: on the right by an ascending rim bowel, colon ascendens, on the left by the root of mesentery, radix mesenterii, and from above by a transverse colon, *colon transversum.* The left mesenteric sine is limited: on the left – by the descending rim bowel, *colon descendens,* on the right – by the obliquely going root of mesentery, *radix mesenterii,* and from below – by a sigmoid bowel, *colon sigmoideum.*

There are two channels in an abdominal region. This channels is located in longitudinal direction. They are right and left lateral channels, *canales longitudinales s. laterales, dexter et sinister.*

The right lateral channel is located between a parietal peritoneum and ascending rim bowel. It extends from the lower surface of the liver to the blind gut. Then it comes behind the cecal eversion. The right lateral channel communicates with hepatic bag near the lower surface of liver.

The left lateral channel is situated between a parietal peritoneum and descending rim bowel. It begins below the left diaphragmatic-rim copula. It stretches downward and between a parietal peritoneum and sigmoid bowel freely reported with the cavity of small pelvis.

Recessus duodenojejunalis is a duodenal-jejunal pocket. It locates between two folds of peritoneum *plica duodenojejunalis superior and plica duodenojejunalis inferior.* Deepening is formed within the limits of *flexura duodenojejunalis* between these folds. This deepening names a duodenal-jejunal pocket. A lower mesenteric vein is located in an upper fold, v. *mesenterica inferior.*

Recessus iliocaecalis superior is an upper iliac-cecal pocket. It is located in an upper corner between an iliac and blind bowel. It is limited above by the iliac-rim fold, *plica iliocolica*. It is limited below by the horizontally going final part of iliac bowel. It is limited outwards by the initial department of the ascending rim bowel, *colon ascendens.*

Recessus iliocaecalis inferior is the lower iliac-cecal pocket. It is a deepening, which is located below the distal part of iliac bowel. The limits of pocket are: above – an iliac bowel, behind – the mesentery of vermicular appendix, *mesentercolum processus appendicularis*, at the front – the iliac-cecal fold of peritoneum, *plica iliocaecalis*, which stretched between distal part iliac and blind bowels.

Clinical value. Accumulations of pathological liquids, which appears in a right sinus, in the beginning limited to the limits of this sinus. The left sinus is open in the cavity of the small pelvis on the down. It does possible distribution of pus or blood. Inflammatory processes can spread on the left and right lateral channels. Pockets are the places of formation of internal hernia. The right hepatic bag is the place of localization of the subphrenic abscess.

Abdominal Cavity Organs (Figures 45, 46)

Abdominal part of gullet extends from the gullet opening of the diaphragm to the cardia opening of the stomach. There are mezo- and intraperitoneal locations in relation to the peritoneum. The arterial blood supply of the gullet carried out from *a. gastrica sinistra* and *aa. phrenicae inferiores.* A portacaval anastomosis is formed. A venous outflow carried out through *v. coronaria ventriculi*. Innervation of esophagus carried out by system of vagus and from a sympathetic frontier barrel. These networks form esophagus interlacement, *plexus esophageus.*

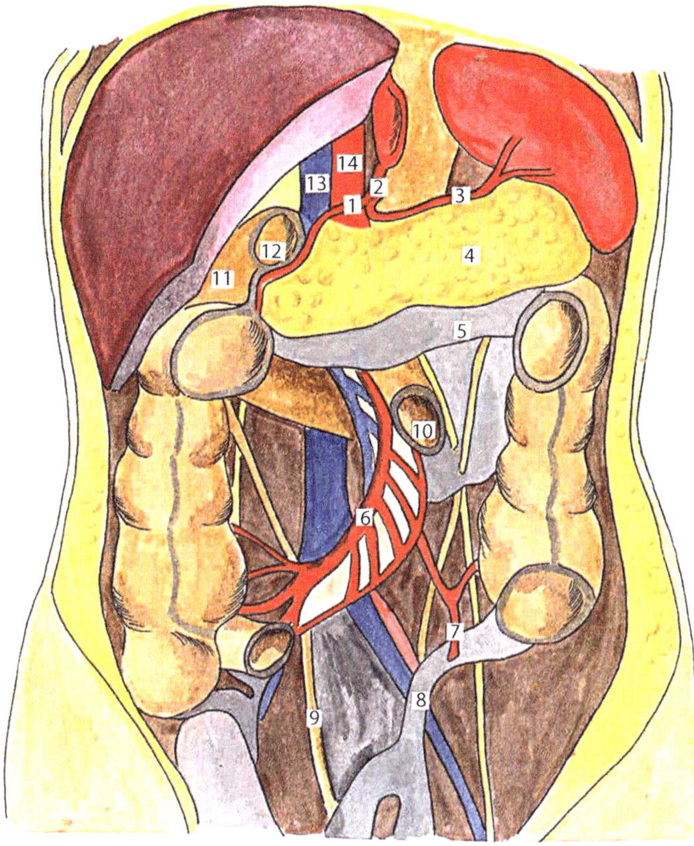

Figure 45 Syntopy of abdominal organs.
1– truncus coeliacus; 2 – a. gastrica dextra; 3 – a. lienalis; 4 – pancreas; 5 – colon transversum mesocolica; 6 – vasa mesenterica superior; 7 – a. sigmoidea; 8 – colon sigmoideun mesocolica; 9 – ureter dexter; 10 – initial of jejunum;11 – pars descendens duodeni; 12 – pars superior horizontalis duodeni; 13 – v. cava inferior; 14 – a. abdominalis.

Esophagus. An esophagus has a funnel-shaped form for children of early age. Its length makes a 10 cm for a newborn. Its length makes a 12 cm for the children of 1 year. Its length makes 18 cm in children of 10 years. The diameter is according to 7–8, 10 and 12–15 mm.

Stomach, *ventriculus* (**Figure 47**). There are *paries anterior* and *paries posterior*, *curvatura minor* and *curvatura major* and five departments: entrance part (*pars cardiaci ventriculi*), bottom (*fundus ventriculi*),

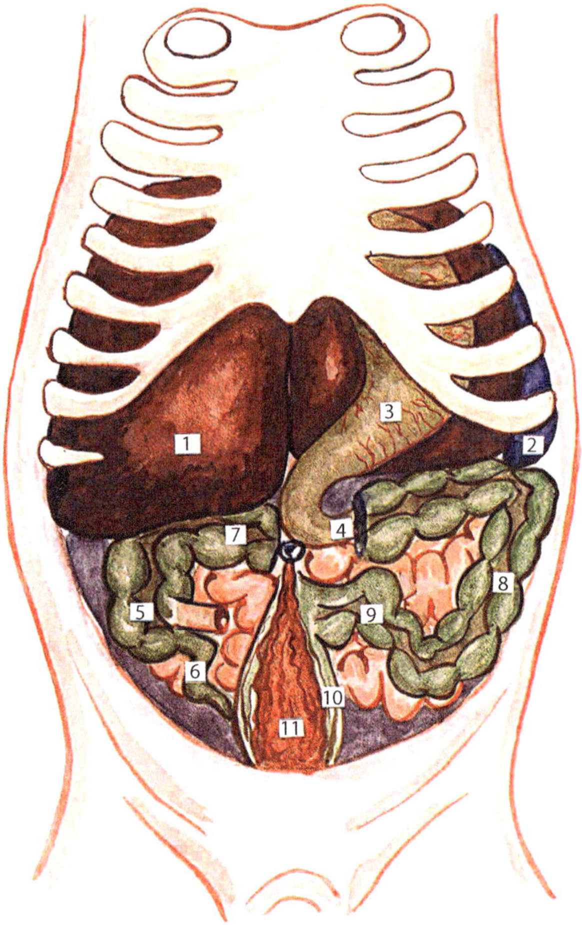

Figure 46 Holotopy of abdominal organs in newborns.
1 – hepar; 2 – lien; 3 – gaster; 4 – duodenum; 5 – caecum; 6 – appendix vermiformis; 7 – colon transversum; 8 – colon descendens; 9 – colon sigmoideum; 10 – rectum; 11 – vesica urinaria.

body of stomach (*corpus ventriculi*), pre-pyloric part (*pars praepylorica*), pyloric part (*pars pylorica*) in it. Distinguish three functional departments of the stomach : secretory, excretory, and incretory.

Three basic variants of the position of the stomach are distinguished. They are slanting, horizontal, and vertical. *Syntopy.* The liver and diaphragm are adjacent to it from above. The *colon transversum* are adjacent to it from below. It is adjacent to the front abdominal wall and also to the lower surface of the left lobe of liver at the front. It is adjacent to

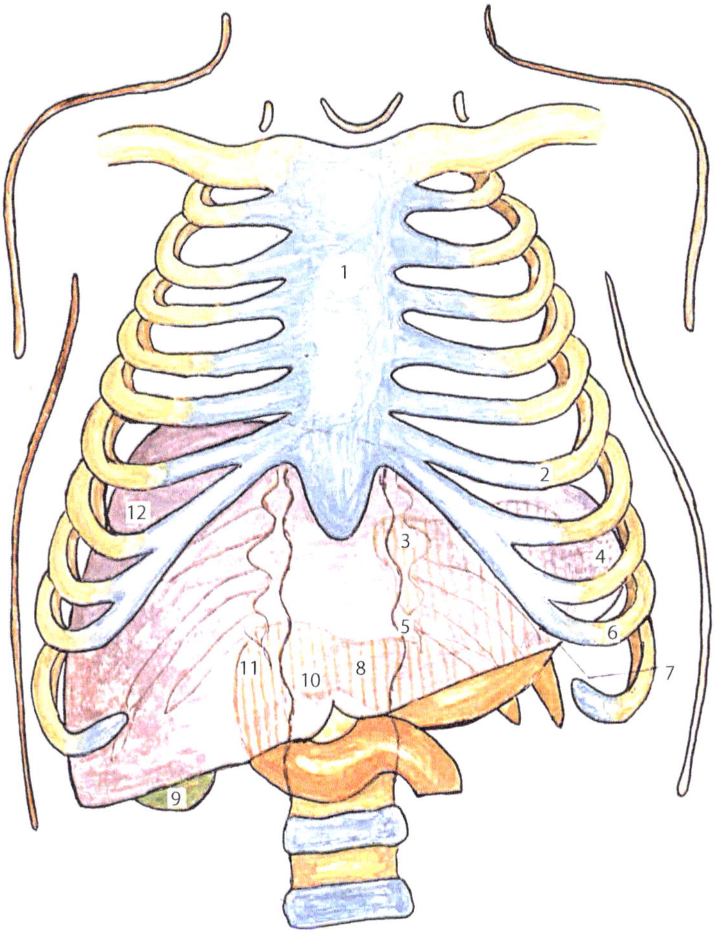

Figure 47 The projection of the liver and stomach to the anterior abdominal wall.
1 – sternum; 2 – costa VIII; 3 – ostium cardiacum ventriculi; 4 –lobus hepatis sinister; 5 – curvatura ventriculi minor; 6 – costa XI; 7 – curvature ventriculi major; 8 – pylorus; 9 – vesica fellea; 10 –fissure lig. teretis; 11 –duodenum; 12 – lobus hepatis dexter.

the organs of retroperitoneal space, to the pancreas, vessels of splenic , to the upper pole of the left bud and to the left adrenal gland behind. The spleen is adjacent to it on the left. The gall-bladder is adjacent to it on the right. The front wall of the stomach is subdivided into two fields. It is depending from abutting to it the same kinds of organs. The upper half of the front part of stomach is covered by the left lobe of the liver. Lower half of gatekeeper is covered by the right lobe of liver.

The upper half of the front wall of the stomach and the lower area of gatekeeper was given the name of the hepatic field of stomach, *area hepatica ventriculi*, for this reason.

Superficial ligamentum of stomach. 1) *lig. gastrocolicum* is a gastrocolic copula; 2) *lig. gastrolienale* is a stomach-splenic copula; 3) *lig. gastrophrenicum* is a gastrophrenic copula; 4) *lig. phrenicoesophageum* is a diaphragmatic-gullet copula; 5) *lig. hepatogastricum* is a hepatogastric copula; 6) *lig. hepatopyloricum* is a hepatopyloric copula.

Deep ligamentum of stomach. 1) *lig. gastropancreaticum* is a gastrointestinal pancreas copula; 2) *lig. pyloropancreaticum* is a pyloric-pancreas copula. A stomach is an intraperitoneal organ.

Blood supply (Figures 48–52). *A. gastrica sinistra* (walks away from *truncus coeliacus*), a. *gastrica dextra* (is a branch of *a. hepatica communis*), *a. gastroepiploica dextra* (is a branch of *a. gastroduodenalis*), *a. gastroepiploica sinistra* (is a branch from *a. lienalis*), *aa. gastrica brevis* (*a. lienalis*).

A venous outflow from a stomach carried out through the system of janitrix. The coronal vein of the stomach located on small curvature of the stomach. v. coronariaventriculi. The second venous vessel of small curvature is the pyloric vein. This vein is directed from the angular notch of the stomach to the area of gatekeeper from left to right.

Innervation. Innervation carried out from the celiac interlacement through the upper and lower stomach, the hepatic, the splenic and upper mesenteric interlacements. The parasympathetic fibres go in composition of left and right wandering barrels. A front (left) wandering trunk (*tractus vagalis anterior*) lies on the front surface of the abdominal department of the gullet. It gives front gastric branches near of stomach. The front branch of small curvature or the front nerve of Latarzhe is the most considerable from the front branches of gastric. It goes to the piloroantralnomu department of the stomach. Except for the front branch of small curvature, the hepatic and the pyloric branches move away from a front trunk. A back (right) wandering

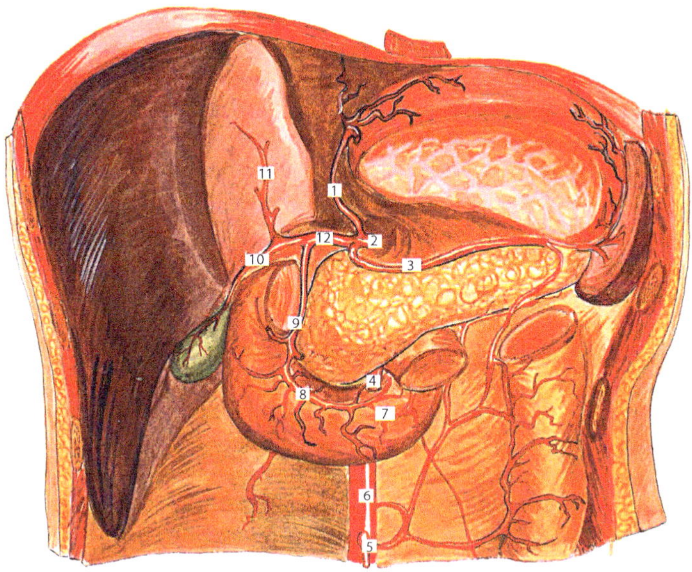

Figure 48 Arteries of the upper abdomen.
1 – a. gastrica sinistra; 2 – truncus celiacus; 3 – a. lienalis; 4 –a. mesenterica superior; 5 –a. mesenterica inferior; 6 – aorta abdominalis; 7 – a. pancreaticoduodenalis inferior; 8 – a. pancreaticoduodenalis superior; 9 – a. gastroduodenalis; 10 – r. a. hepaticae dexter; 11 – r. a. hepaticae sinister; 12 –.a. hepatica communis.

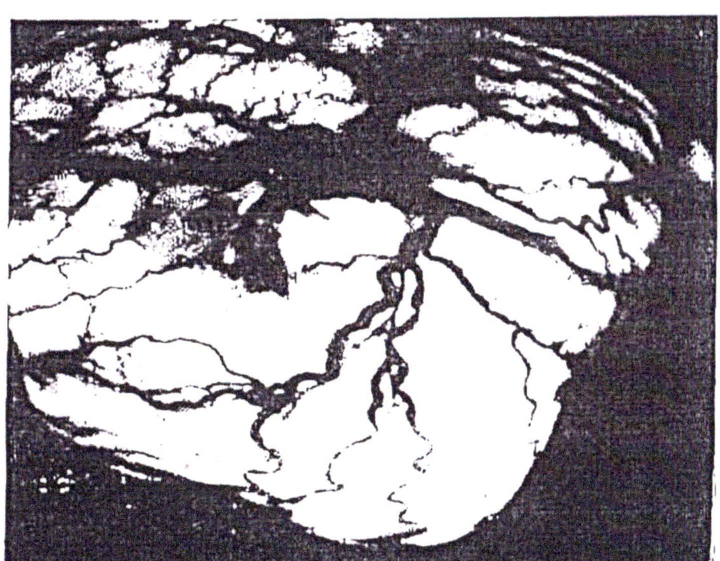

Figure 49 Vessels submucosal plexus of the fundus (transillumination angiography).

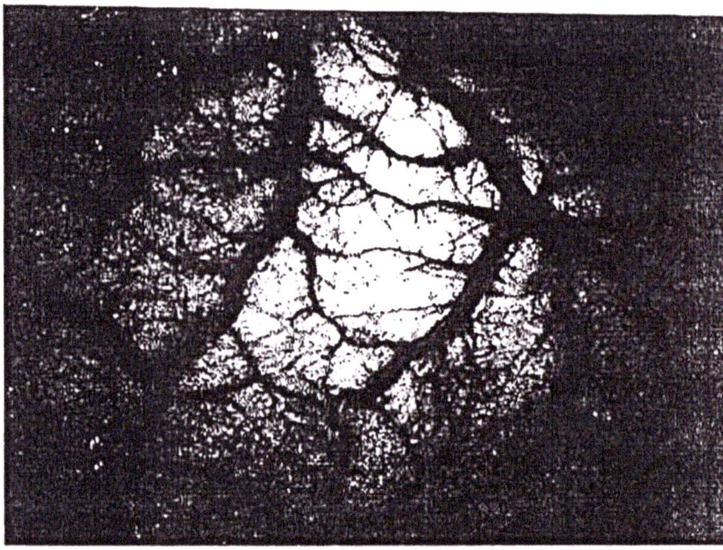

Figure 50 Anastomoses between intramural vessels submucosal plexus of the anterior wall of the stomach, which entering into the stomach wall from the small and large curvature.

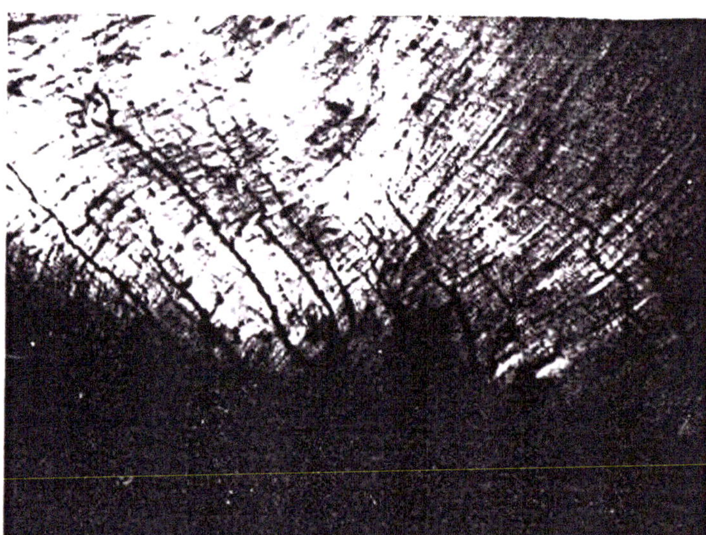

Figure 51 The serous-muscular layer of the stomach of the dog in transmitted light.

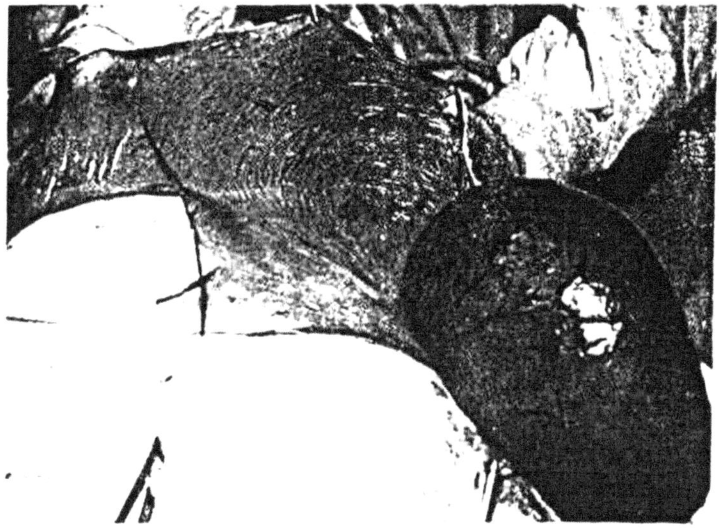

Figure 52 The digested stomach reflected light (experiment on dogs).

trunk (*tractus vagalis posterior*) lies between the back surface of gullet and abdominal aorta after an exit from the oesophageal opening of diaphragm. It gives back branches of gastric, including the back nerve of small curvature. Sympathetic fibres form two interlacements. They are upper and lower stomach. The upper stomach interlacements is situated along the left artery of stomach. The lower stomach interlacements accompanies a gastroduodenal artery.

Anomalies of development. The complete and incomplete doubling of stomach, partial narrowing of antral department, congenita stenosis of gatekeeper, the reverse position of the stomach, "pectoral stomach", the congenita giantism of folds, cardiospasm, pyloristenosis. The stomach has the rounded, some prolate form in the newborn. It is located in the left infracostal area. It is located horizontally in most cases. It is covered by the left stake of liver in front. The pyloric part is situated in a sagital plane near from the gate of liver.

A duodenum is subdivided into four departments. It is an upper horizontal part, *pars horizontalis superior*, the descending part, *pars* *descendens*, the lower horizontal part, *pars horizontalis inferior,* and the ascending part, *pars ascendens*. The covering its peritoneum is the back wall of cavity of epiploon. There are three copulas of the duodenum: 1) *lig. hepatoduodenale*; 2) *lig. suspensorium duodeni*; 3) *lig. duodenorenale.*

Skeletopy. The duodenum is situated on the different height of backbone. It is situated behind a stomach most often. The upper horizontal part is situated at the level of the 1st lumbar vertebra usually. This part of the bowel crosses a middle plane in transversal direction from left to right. It begins from the gatekeeper of the stomach. The descending part of the bowel fits closely to the right surfaces of lumbar vertebrae. It extends from top down to the lower 3th lumbar vertebra. A horizontal lower part lies at the level of the 3th lumbar vertebra. It crosses its middle plane from right to left in transversal direction. The ascending part crosses from the left of body of the lumbar vertebra to the left surface of its body to the level of 2nd lumbar vertebra on the left, where this part of duodenum becomes to the jejunum (*intestinum jejunum*) after formation of duodenal-jejunal bend (*fiexura duodenojejunalis*).

Syntopy (Figures 53, 54). *Pars horizontalis superior duodeni.* Next organs adjoin this department of the duodenum. Above there is a gallbladder and *lig. hepatoduodenale*; below there is a head of pancreas and part of body of pancreas; in front there is an antral part of the stomach; behind there is backbone. *Pars descendens duodeni* is surrounded by next organs. In front there are loops of thin bowels; behind – is a back wall of cavity of stomach (ribs, intercostal muscles); outside – is the right kidney with part of ureter. The duodenum is the retroperitoneal organ. It is fortified in the retroperitoneum motionlessly.

Blood supply. The arterial supply of duodenum is carried out from two sources: by system of the celiac artery and by the upper mesenteric artery, *a. mesenterica superior.* Blood enters in the upper pancreatic-duodenal artery, *a. pancreaticoduodenalis superior,* from the first system through the general hepatic artery, *a. hepatica communis,*

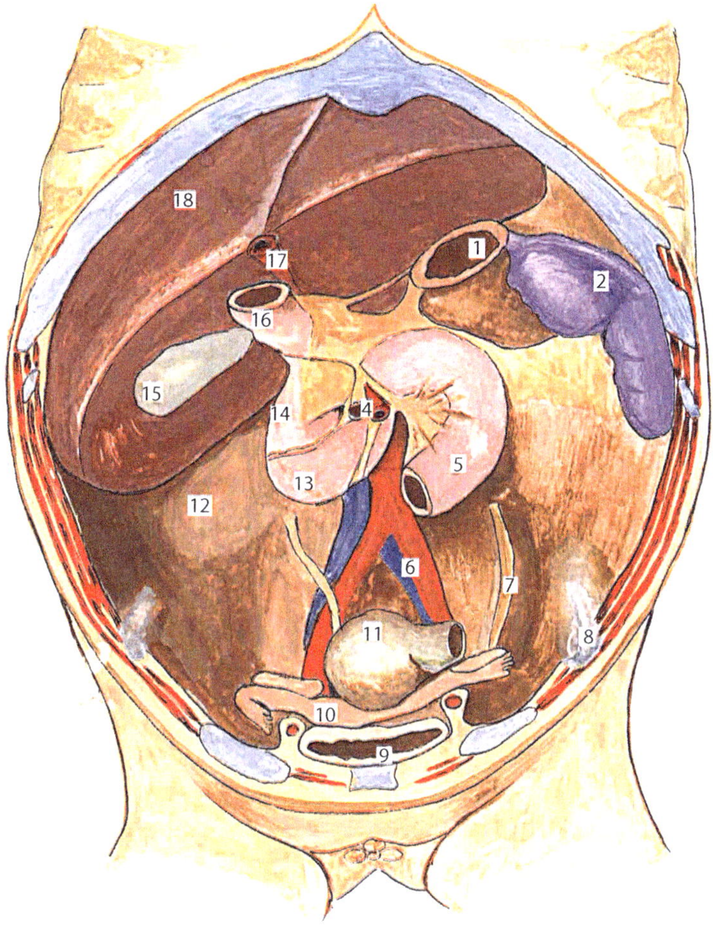

Figure 53 The topography of the duodenum.
1 – ostium cardiacum ventriculi; 2 – lien; 3 – pancreas; 4 – vasa mesenterica superior; 5 – jejunum; 6 – vasa iliaca communis; 7 – ureter sinister; 8 – spina iliaca anterior superior; 9 – vesica urinaria; 10 – uterus; 11 – rectum; 12 – ren dexter; 13 – pars horizontalis duodeni; 14 – pars descendens duodeni; 15 – vesica fellea; 16 – pylorus; 17 – v. umbilicalis; 18 – lobus hepatis dexter.

the gastroduodenal artery, *a. gastroduodenalis*. In the system of upper mesenteric artery, *a. mesenterica superior*, blood supply is carried out from the lower pancreatic- duodenal artery, *a. pancreaticoduodenalis inferior*. Both indicated vessels form the same name arterial arch, *arcus arteriosus pancreaticoduodenalis*. This arch is located in a front pancreatic-duodenal groove, *sulcus pancreaticoduodenalis anterior*.

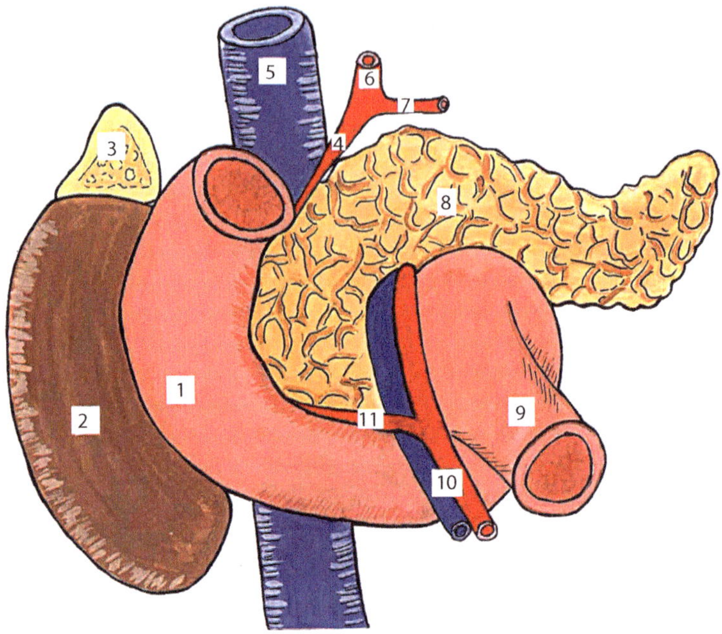

Figure 54 Syntopy of the duodenum and pancreas.
1 – duodenum; 2 – ren dexter; 3 – suprarenalis dexter; 4 – a. pancreaticoduodenalis superior; 5 – v. cava inferior; 6 – a. gastroduodenalis; 7 – a. gastroepiploitica dextra; 8 – pancreas; 9 – the beginning of the jejunum; 10 – a. et v. mesenterica superior; 11 – a. pancreaticoduodenalis inferior.

Innervation. The duodenum is innervated from the branches that begin in the upper mesenteric interlacement, *plexus mesenterica superior*. These branches contain sympathetic fibres. The pancreatic-duodenal branches move away from the mesenteric interlacement, *rami pancreaticoduodenales*. These branches are accompanied by the same name arterial vessels, *aa. pancreaticoduodenales*. These branches penetrate into the head of pancreas and the duodenum wall.

Anomalies of development are the partial narrowing of road clearance, atresia, the congenita stenosis, webbed membrane fusion, arteriomezenterialnaya obstruction, the acute duodenal obstruction arteriomezenterialnaya, doubling, duplication cyst, compression of duodenum, anomalies of location of duodenum.

The duodenum is situated at the level of 12th thoracal or 1st lum bar vertebrae in the newborn. The upper horizontal part of bowel is covered by a liver. A general bilious duct, janitrix and hepatic artery are located behind the duodenum. Below there is a head of pancreas. The descending part of bowel is covered by a liver also. The ascending part of the rim bowel adjoins it from a lateral side. The medial department of the right adrenal adjoins it behind. The upper mesenteric vessels pass at front from ascending part of the bowel.

Thin bowel (*intestinum tenue*) **(Figure 55).** The *duodenum, intestinum jejunum, intestinum ilium* belong to the thin bowel.

Root of mesentery (**Figure 56**), *radix mesenterii*, corresponds to the left surface of body of 2nd lumbar vertebrae. There is *plica duodenojejunalis* in this place. The root of mesentery goes downward and to the right, crosses a backbone and ends at *articulatio sacroiliaca dextra* from here. The distinctive signs of jejunum from iliac consist in a presence on the mucous membrane of jejunum of numerous half-round folds, *plicae circulares*. To the iliac bowel is peculiar a presence of a lot of solitary follicles *folliculi solitarii* and Peyer's name-plates.

Projection is a celiac and hypogastric to the area of front wall of the stomach.

Syntopy. Organs of retroperitoneal space are located behind the thin bowel. The transverse colon and its mesentery are located above the thin bowel. Loops of bowel lie between a sigmoid and direct bowel behind and by a urinary bladder at the front from below for men. Loops of bowel lie between a sigmoid and direct bowel behind and by a uterus from below for women. A blind gut, vermicular appendix, the ascending rim of bowel lie on the right. An ascending rim of bowel lies on the left.

Blood supply: a. mesenterica superior, a. pancreaticoduodenalis inferior, a. colica media et dextra, a. ileocolica, aa. jejunales et aa. ilei.

Innervation. *plexus mesentericus superior.*

Colon (*intestinum crassum*).

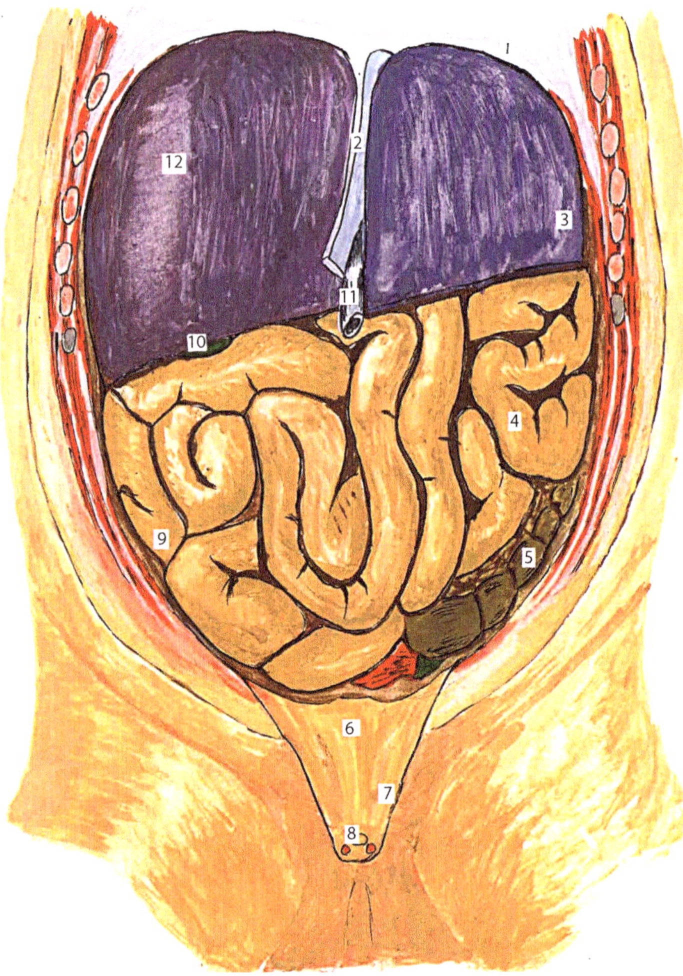

Figure 55 Organs of the abdominal cavity. Anterior abdominal wall of the stomach is removed.
1 – diaphragma; 2 – lig. falciforme hepatic; 3 – lobus hepatis sinister; 4 – intestinum tenue; 5 – colon sigmoideum; 6 – vesica urinaria; 7 – plica umbilicalis medialis; 8 – urachus; 9 – ileum; 10 – vesica fellea; 11 – v. umbilicalis; 12 – lobus hepatis dexter.

Blind gut, *intestlnum caecum*, is the initial segment of thick bowels. It is situated below the place of confluence of iliac bowel in colon. There are four morphological variations of blind gut: cone-shaped, saccate, symmetric-bay shaped, asymmetric-shaped bay.

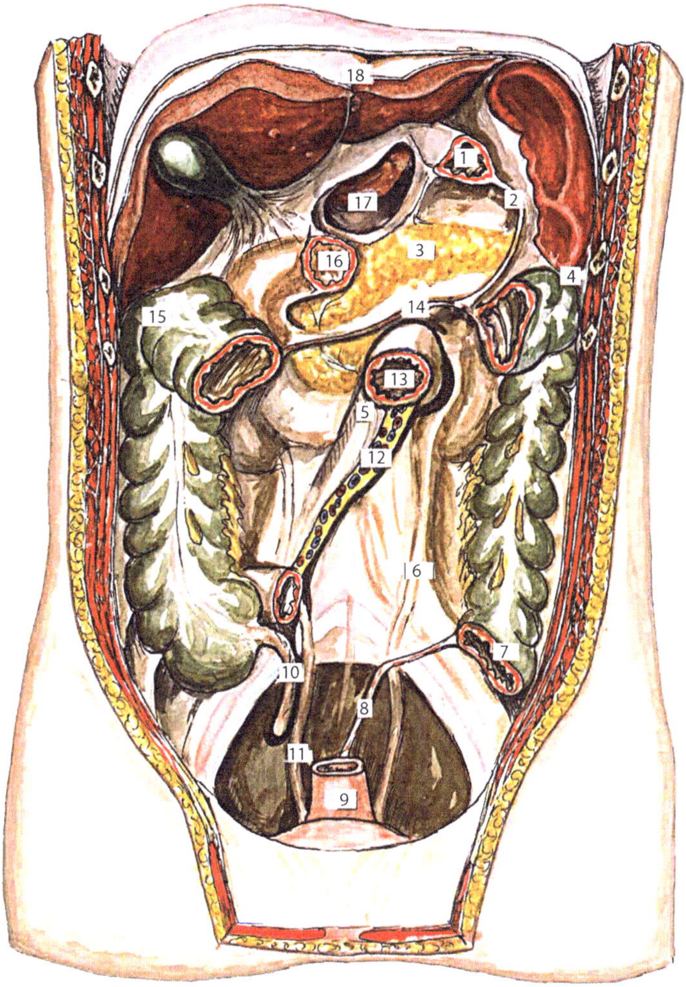

Figure 56 The lines of attachment mesentericof thin intestine and colon.
1 – pars cardiacus ventriculi; 2 – lig. gastrolienale; 3 – pancreas; 4 – lig. phrenicocolicum; 5 –pars ascendens duodeni; 6 – ureter sinister (relief); 7 – colon sigmoideum; 8 – mesosigmoideum; 9 – rectum; 10 – appendix; 11 – ureter dexter (relief); 12 – radix mesenterii; 13 – flexura duodenojejunalis; 14 – mesenterium coli transversi; 15 – flexura intestine crassi dextra; 16 – pars superior duodeni; 17 – omentum minus; 18 – lig. falciforme hepatis.

The place of position of blind gut corresponds to the right iliac fossula, *fossa iliaca dextra*, in ordinary terms. The length of the blind gut is approximately equal to its width and varies in limits from 6 to 8 cm.

laterally. All its parts are located mezoperitoneally except the upper and lower ends. There is a short mesentery only next to *flexura coli sinistra*, and also in the place of its becoming to *colon sigmoideum*. The descending rim bowel is situated in a furrow between *m. psoas major* and *m. transversus abdominis*. It fits closely behind to *m.quadratus lumborum*.

A sigmoid bowel, *colon sigmoideum*, begins approximately at the level of crista iliaca. It extends to the border between the 2nd and 3th of a sacrum vertebra. A mesanteric of sigmoid bowel, *mesosigmoideum,* ends at this level. The sigmoid bowel comes at first to mezoperitoneal position, and then to the extraperitoneal one. The lower end of *mesosigmoideum* is a border between a sigmoid and direct bowel. The position of sigmoid bowel varies depending on the degree of filling of both bowel and nearby pelvic organs. The sigmoid bowel goes down in a small pelvis at an empty line bowel and urinary bladder.

Projection of colon. Blind gut, vermicular appendix are projected in the right iliac area of the front wall of the stomach. The ascending rim bowel is projected in the right lateral area. The hepatic curvature of the rim bowel is projected in the right subcostal. The transversal rim bowel is projected in the umbilical area. The splenic curvature of rim bowel is projected in the left subcostal. The descending rim bowel is projected in the left lateral area. The sigmoid bowel is projected in the left iliac and suprapubic area. The founding of the vermicular appendix is projected in the point of Lanza.

Blood supply of bowels (Figures 58, 59). All bowels are supplied by the mesenteric arteries, except the initial department of duodenum.

A.mesenterica superior is an upper mesenteric artery. It moves away from the aorta at the level of the 1st lumbar vertebra. It is subdivided into two parts: the pancreas posterior part, *pars retropancreatica*, and duodenal-jejunal part, *pars duodenoieliinalis*. The branches of upper mesenteric artery are:

1. *A. pancreaticoduodenalis inferior* is the lower pancreatic-duodenum artery. It departs at the level of the upper edge

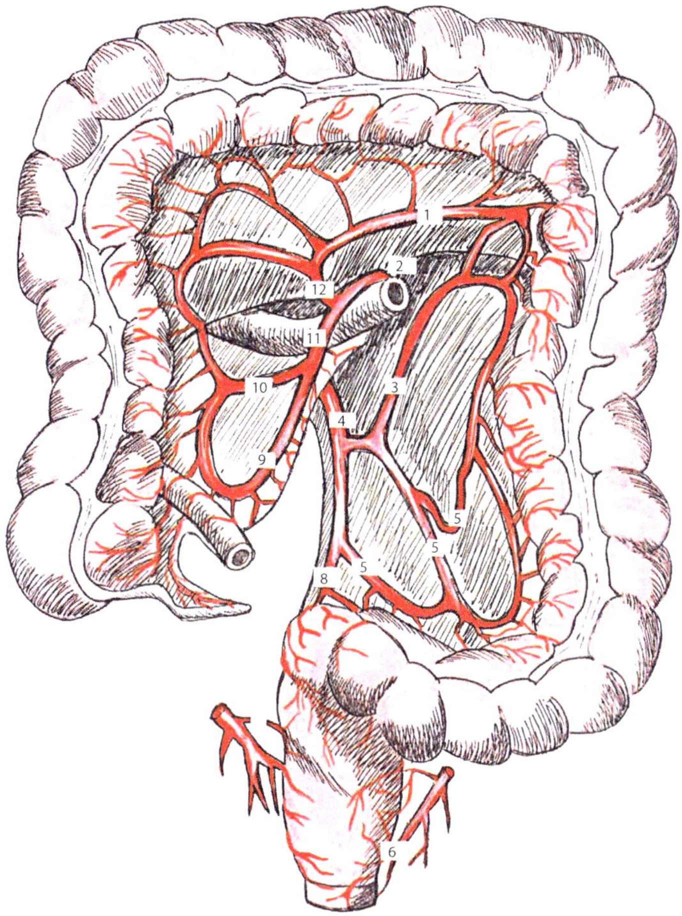

Figure 58 Blood supply of the colon.
1 – anastomosis a. colica media et a. colica sinistra; 2 – plica duodenojejunalis; 3 – a. colica sinistra; 4 – a. mesenterica inferior; 5 – a. sigmoidea; 6 – a. rectalis inferior; 7 – a. rectalis media; 8 – a. rectalis superior; 9 – a. iliaca et colon ascendens; 10 – a. colica dextra; 11 – a. mesenterica superior; 12 – a. colica media.

of horizontal part of duodenum and goes up, lies down in a furrow between the head of the pancreas and horseshoe of duodenum (*sulcus pancreaticoduodenalis*). The artery anastomoses with an upper pancreatic-duodenum artery, *a. pancreaticoduodenalis superior*, and forms a pancreatic-duodenum arterial arc, *arcus arteriosus pancreaticoduodenalis*, when rising up.

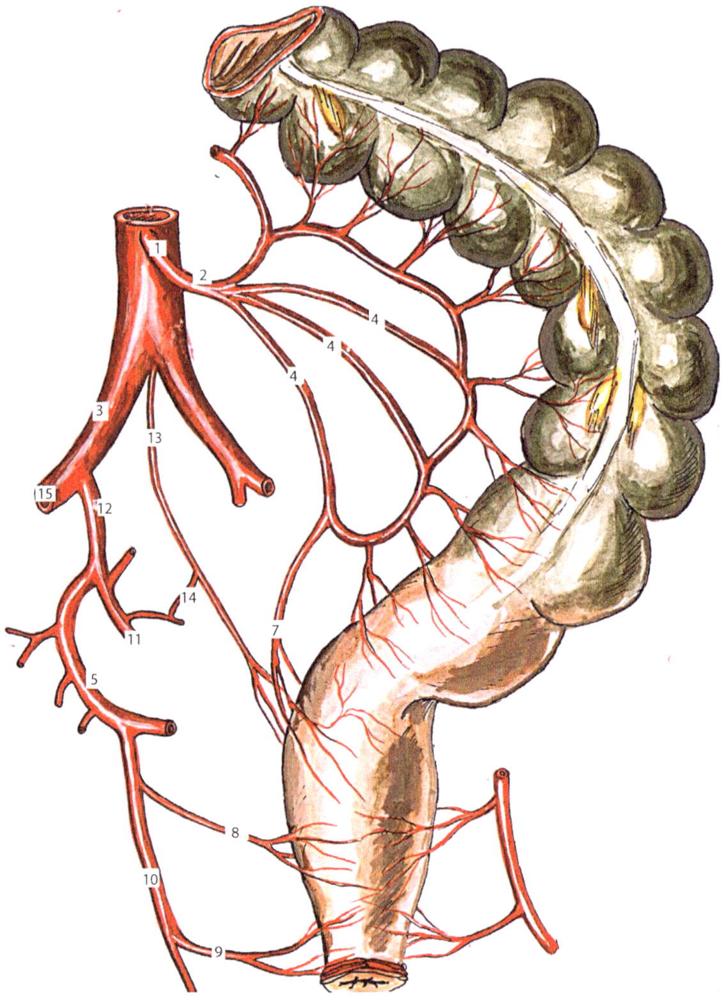

Figure 59 Blood supply of the sigmoid colon and rectum.
1 – a. mesenterica inferior; 2 – a. colica sinistra; 3 – a. iliaca communis; 4 – aa. sigmoideae; 5 – r. anterior a. iliaca interna; 6 – aorta; 7 – a. rectalis superior; 8 – a. rectalis media; 9 – a. rectalis inferior; 10 – a. pudenda interna; 11 – a. glutea superior; 12 –a. iliaca interna; 13 – a. sacralis media; 14 – anastomosis a. sacralis medialis et lateralis; 15 – a. iliaca externa.

2. *Rami intestinales* are intestinal branches. They are directed to the left and supplied with blood of jejunal loop (*rami jejunales*) and iliac loop (*rami iliaci*) bowels. *A. ileocolica* is an iliac-rim artery. It moves away from the right semicircle of the upper mesenteric artery and directed to the

blind gut. It is subdivided into the three eventual branches: *ramus appendicularis* is the branch of vermicular appendix , which is located in its mesenteric; *ramus iliacus* is an iliac branch, it supplied with blood final part (*pars terminalis*) of iliac bowel; *ramus colicus* is a rim branch, it feeds a blind gut, near to blind gut.

3. *A. colica dextra* is a right rim artery. It departs higher than previous and is supplied with blood *colon ascendens*. It anastomoses with a overlying middle rim artery.

4. *A. colica media* is a middle rim artery. It moves also away from the right semicircle of the artery over of *a. colica dextra*. It gives a descending branch and ascending branch. The descending branch anastomosis with a *a. colica dextra*. The ascending branch forms the wide arched anastomosis with a *a. colica sinistra*.

A. mesenterica superior supplied with blood pancreas through the a. *pancreaticoduodenalis inferior* also.

A. mesenterica inferior is a lower mesenteric artery. It begins from an aorta at the level of lumbar vertebra. It is located in the left mesenteric sine after than of intestinal loops throw to the right. The artery is subdivided into final branches, when is directed to the left iliac fossa.

1. *A. colica sinistra* is the left rim artery. It is supplied with blood the left part of *colon transversum* and all *colon descendens*.

2. *A. sigmoidea* is a sigmoid artery. It is directed in the number of 2–3 branches and provides with blood the sigmoid bowel.

3. *A. rectalis superior* is an upper rectal artery. It is the final branch of *a. mesenterica superior*. It is directed to the small pelvis, is bent through *promontorium* and branches out in

the upper department of rectum. It anastomoses with a *a. sigmoidea*, and with a *a. rectalis media*.

A venous outflow is carried out from the unpaired abdominal cavity organs to the system of janitrix. The blood of pair organs of abdomen cavity, buds and adrenals is carried out by the system of postcava.

V. portae is a janitrix. It is located behind the head of the pancreas. Three veins take part in its formation:

- Coronary vein of the stomach, v. coronaria ventriculi, goes along a small curvature from left to right, on the way taking branches from the ventral part of the esophagus and cardia. Within the gatekeeper, it anastomoses with the pyloric veins, v. pyloricae. It flows more often into the portal vein directly, rarely – into the superior mesenteric vein.

- Cystic vein, v. cystica, accompanies the same artery and lies in the wall of the gallbladder. Driving from the bottom to the neck of the gallbladder, the cystic vein flows into the right branch of the portal vein.

- Upper mesenteric vein, *v. mesenterica superior*, passes directly above the main trunk of the portal vein, accompanying the same artery on the right side. It rises up in an oblique direction, lying in the root of the mesentery, and in its way accepts the veins of the small intestines, *vv. Intestinales*, vein of jejunum and ileum, *vv. jeunales et ileales*, right and medial sciatic veins, *vv. colicae dextra et media*; ilio-colon vein, v. ileocolica; pancreatic veins, *vv. pancreaticae*; vein of the appendix, v.appendicularis, pancreas-duodenal veins, *vv. pancreaticoduodenalis*; right gastro-omental vein, *v. gastroepiploica dextra*; splenic vein, *v. lienalis*, which is the second most significant inflow of the portal vein; carries blood from the spleen and accepts short gastric veins, *vv. gastricae breves*, from the bottom of the stomach and left gastro-omental vein, *v. gastroepiploica sinistra,* pancreatic veins, *vv. pancreaticae.*

- Lower mesenteric vein, *v. mesenterica inferior*, accompanies the same artery. It is formed by the upper rectal vein, *v. rectalis superior*, S-shaped veins, *vv. sigmoideae*, and left colonic vein, *v. colica sinistra.*

The trunk of the portal vein has the length of about 5cm. The vein is deprived of valves and formed behind the pancreas head. It is formed due to confluence of v. mesenterica superior and v. lienalis.

Features of blood supply in children (**Figure 60).**

Innervation. Sympathetic frontier trunks, vagal and diaphragmatic nerves, take part in the supply of organs of the abdominal cavity. These nerves form vast interlacements. These interlacements present the peripheral department of the nervous system. The following vegetative interlacements of the abdominal cavity are distinguished: *plexus aorticus abdominalis* is an abdominal aortic interlacement, it as a wide network which is situated on an abdominal aorta, it widely anastomases with other adjoining interlacements; *Plexus solaris* is sunny interlacement, it is the largest vegetative interlacement of the body and is presented by two large lunate ganglies, *ganglia semilunaria,* fitting to each side of the aorta at the level of departing *a. coeliaca.* The wide network of nerve plexus anastomoses with mesenteric plexus lying below.

The sunny interlacement is composed of several nervous networks that accompany corresponding vessels. It is *plexus phrenicus,* diaphragmatic interlacement. It is located in the adventitia of *a. phrenica inferior. Plexus hepaticus* is a hepatic interlacement. It is unpaired. It is located along the *a. hepatica* and widely anostomoses with the upper and lower gastric interlacements. *Plexus gastricus superior* is an upper gastric interlacement. It is unpaired also; it is located on the small curvature of the stomach. It is coonected with the branches of vagal, diaphragmatic nerves. *Plexus gastricus inferior* is a lower gastric interlacements. It accompanies the same name artery and gives branches

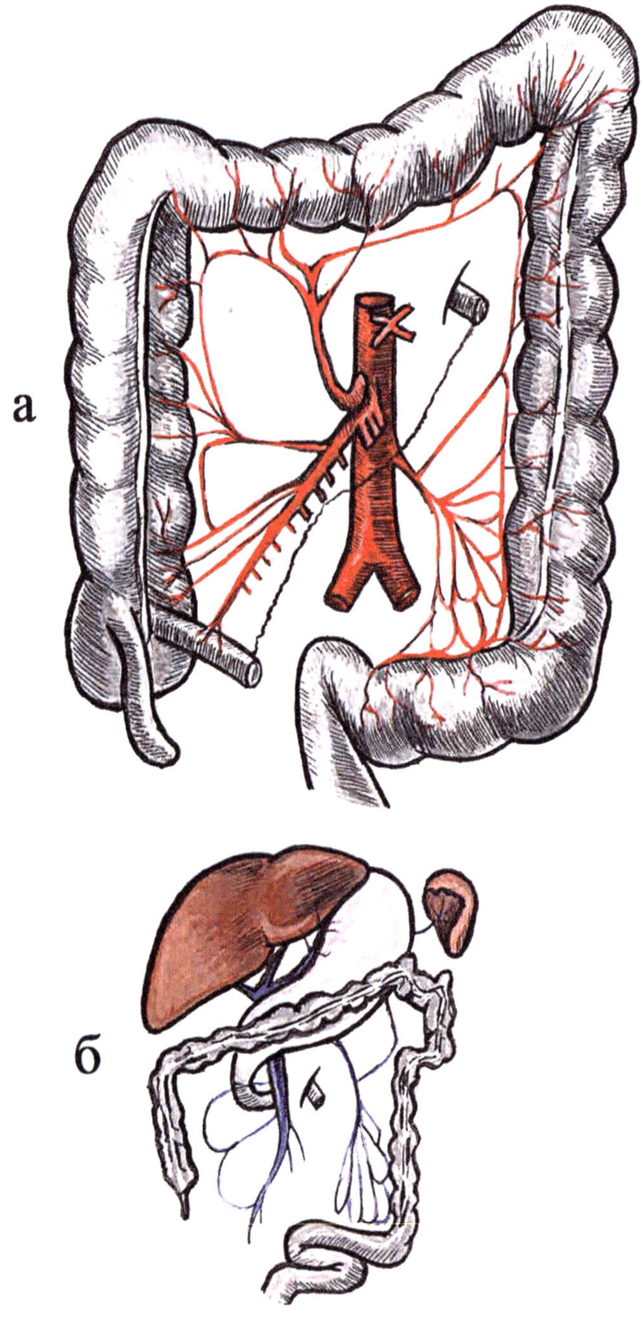

Figure 60 Features of the blood supply of the large intestine in the newborn: a, b - a typical anatomical diagram of the main arteries (a) and veins (b) of the colon.

to the pancreas and spleen. *Plexus suprarenalis* is an adrenal interlacement. It is a paired interlacement. It accompanies the same-name vessels and innervates the adrenal. *Plexus renalis* is a kidney interlacement. It accompanies kidney vessels; it is a paired interlacement. It anastomoses with *plexus coeliacus* and *plexus mesentericus superior. Plexus spermaticus internus* is an internal seminal interlacement. It is a paired interlacement; it is located in the adventitia of the same name vessels. *Plexus mesentericus superior* is an upper mesenteric interlacement. It is unpaired interlacement. It is a direct continuation of the sunny interlacement that goes downwards. *Plexus mesentericus inferior* is a lower mesenteric interlacement. It is also unpaired. Its branches accompany the same-name artery. It innervates a descending rim, sigmoid bowel and partly an upper department of the rectum. *Plexus hypogastricus* is a hypogastric interlacement. It is a vast sympathetic interlacement of the small pelvis.

Abnomalities of the development: doubling, agenesis segment of intestinal tube, aplasia of mucous membrane, membranous atresia, plural aplasia, megacolon (illness of Hirschsprung), Meckel diverticulum.

Bowels. The bowels are relatively longer in children than in adults. It exceeds the length of body by 6 times in infants. It exceeds the length of body by 4 times in adults. Its absolute length varies individually in large limits. A blind gut and appendix are movable. The appendix is often situated atypically. It complicates diagnostics in an inflammation. Sigmoid bowel is of relatively greater length than in adults. It forms loops in some children. It contributes to the development of primary constipations. A mesentery is longer and easily dilates due to this torsion, invaginations of intestinal loopsin occur.

A liver (Figure 61) is located in the right infracostal area, *regio hypochondrica dextra*, in an anticardium, *scrobiculum cordis*, and its left lobe is partly located in the left infracostal area, *regio hypochondrica sinistra*.

The liver is subdivided into the right and left lobe, *lobus dexter et lobus sinister*. A border between them is sagittally located suspending or falcate copula of liver, *lig. suspensorium*. Extra-peritoneal area, *area*

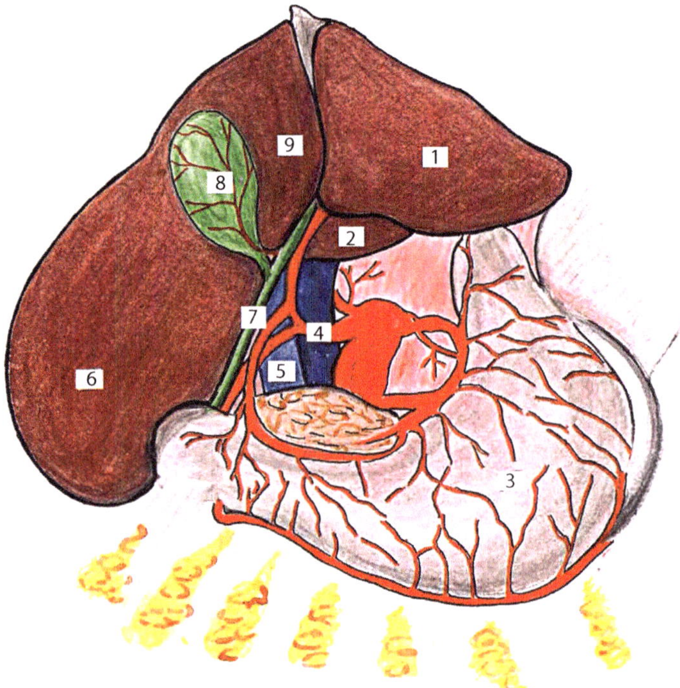

Figure 61 Liver.
1 – lobus hepaticus sinister; 2 – lobus caudatus hepatis; 3 – gaster; 4 – a. hepatica propria; 5 – v. portae; 6 - lobus hepaticus dexter; 7 – ductus choledochus; 8 – vesica fellea; 9 – lobus quadrates hepatis.

hepatis extraperitonealis, adjoins the diaphragm; due to this the level of liver location depends on the height of diaphragm standing. Six organs adjoin the lower surface of the liver (**Figure 62**). They are *colon transversum, ren dexter, glandula suprarenalis, ventriculus, esophagus* and *duodenum*. The back surface of the liver adjoins the lumbar and costal part of diaphragms.

Projection. The part of the liver, which is adherent to the thoracal and abdominal walls, is possible to subdivide into three areas: upper, middle and lower. The upper area is covered by the lower lobe of the right lung. Here in direct injury the pleura cavity is dissected, lung and the upper area of liver are damaged. The middle area is projected behind the lower edge of *sinus phrenicocostalis*. A direct wound in this area gives a dissection to the pleura cavity without damage of the lung and

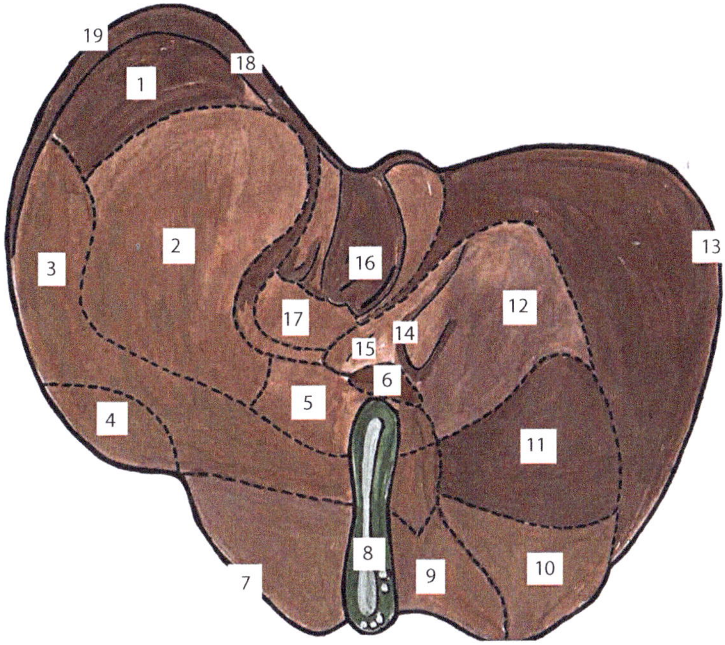

Figure 62 Visceral surface of the liver and its topography.
1 – impression lienalis; 2 – impressio gastrica; 3 – impression colica; 4 – the area, which contacts with the intestinal loops; 5 – impression duodenalis; 6 – lobus caudatus; 7 – margo inferior; 8 – vesica fellea; 9 – the area, which contacts with the intestinal loops; 10 – impression colica; 11 – impressio renalis; 12 – impressio suprarenalis; 13-lobusdexter; 14 – v. portae; 15 – porta hepatis; 16 – lobus cuadratus; 17 – impression pancreatic; 18 -impressio esophagea; 19 – lobus sinister.

middle area of the liver. The lower area of the liver adjoins the front abdominal wall. In an injury only the liver is damaged, without dissection of pleura cavity.

Syntopy (Figure 63). The upper surface of the liver adjoins the diaphragm, the front surface adjoins the diaphragm and front abdominal wall, the back surface adjoins the 10th and 11th pectoral vertebrae, to the legs of diaphragm, abdominal department of gullet, aorta, right adrenal and to *v. cava inferior*. Lower surface adjoins the upper horizontal part of duodenum, *flexura coli dextra* and gall-bladder.

Blood supply. The liver is supplied with the blood from the system of general hepatic artery, *a. hepatica communis*. It is the branch of *a.*

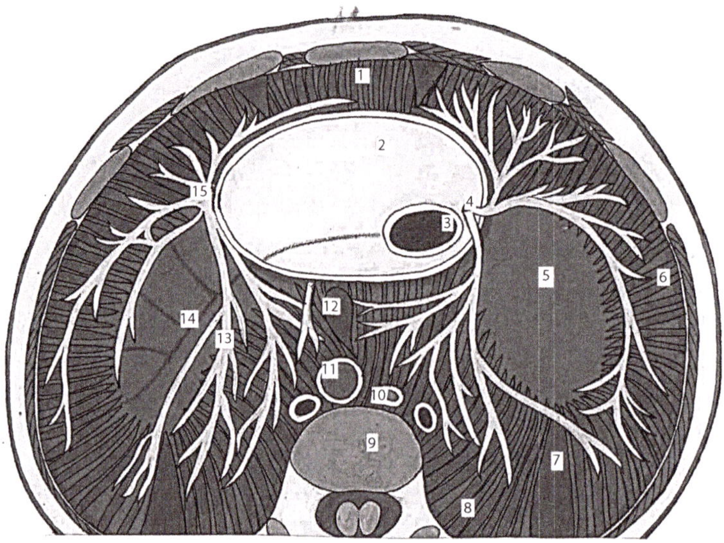

Figure 64 The topography of the nerves of the diaphragm.
1 – diaphragma (pars sternalis); 2 – pericardium (pars diaphragmatica) 3 – v. cava inferior 4 – n. phrenicus dexter 5 – centrum tendineum 6 – diaphragma (pars costalis) 7 – trigonum sternocostale 8 – diaphragma (pars lumbalis); 9 – cartilage intervertebralis 10 – ductus limphaticus 11 – aorta 12 – hiatus esophagealis 13 – r. posterior n. phrenici sinistri 14 – v. phrenica inferior sinistra; 15 – n. phrenicus sinister.

Abnomalities of development: hepatomegalia, hypoplasia of separate lobes of liver, hypoplasia of liver, dystopia of liver, additional lobe of liver.

The liver of newborn (**Figure 66**) occupies from 1/2 to 2/3 volumes of abdominal cavity (The liver occupies 1/3 volume of abdominal cavity in adults). Its surface is smoothed by weakly expressed deepenings of the organs, which adjoin the liver. The left lobe exceeds or equals to the right lobe in its sizes. A gate is more often displaced to the back edge and has the closed type of structure. It is possible to distinguish only basic trunks of the right and left branches of hepatic artery in this type.

Gall-bladder, *cystis s. vesica fellea*, is a reservoir for collecting bile. The gall-bladder is located in the right infracostal area, where it lies in the front department of the right sagittal furrow of the liver (*sulcus segitalis dexter*). The fossula of gall-bladder is formed here. The peritoneal cover covers a gall-bladder unevenly. The bottom of the bladder is located intraperitoneally, and its body and neck are located mezoperitonealy.

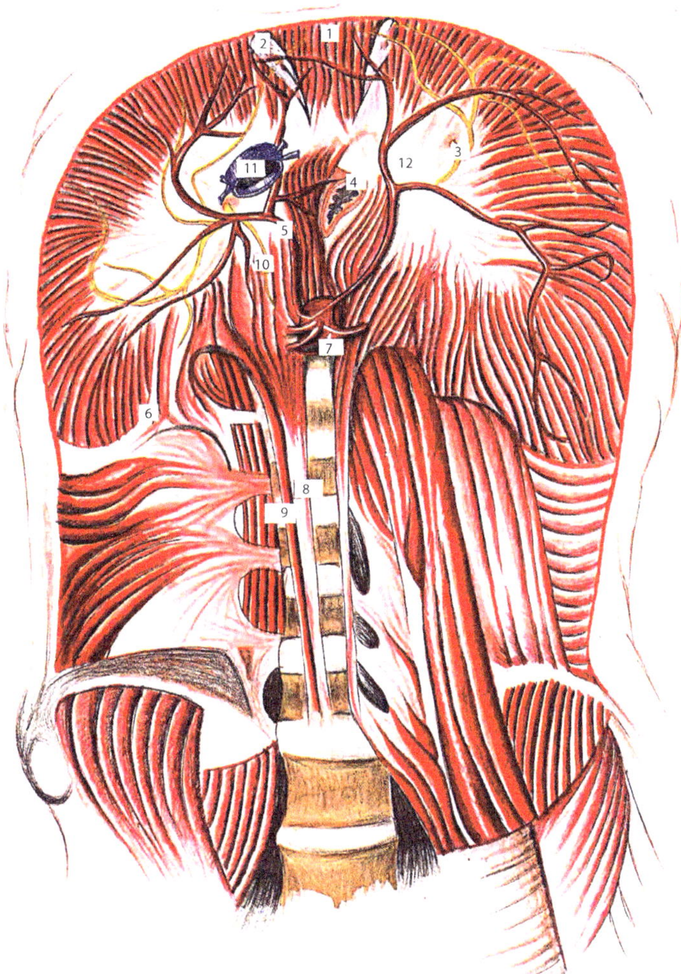

Figure 65 Diaphragma.
1 - pars sternalis diaphragmatic; 2 - trigonum sternocostalis; 3 - n. phrenicus sinister; 4 – esophagus; 5 - a. phrenica dextra; 6 - trigonum lumbocostalis; 7 – aorta (pars abdominalis); 8 – crus dextrum diaphragmatic mediale; 9 - crus dextrum diaphragmatic laterale; 10 - n. phrenicus dexer; 11 - v. cava inferior; 12 - centrum tendineum diaphragmatic.

Projection is a right subcostal area.

Syntopy of gall-bladder: the gall-bladder is covered by the right lobe of the liver upwards, it adjoins *colon transversum* downwards, it touches a gatekeeper and *pars horizontalis superior duodeni* from the inside, *flexura coli dextra* joins to its outside.

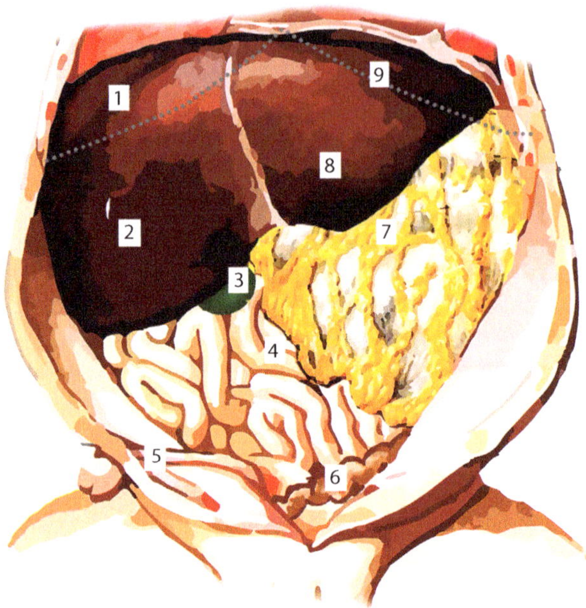

Figure 66 Liver of the newborn. The dashed line indicates the edge of the costal arch.
1 – hepar; 2 – lobus dexter; 3 – vesica fellea; 4 – interstinum tenue; 5 – plica umbilicalis mediana; 6 – S-образная кишка; 7 – omentum majus; 8 – lobus sinistra; 9 – facies diaphragmatica

The blood supply (Figures 67, 68) of the gall-bladder is carried out due to *a. cystica* from the system of *a. hepatica propria*. This vessel has an important surgical value during the operation of gall-bladder removal, *cholecystectomy*.

The identification triangle of Kahlo is used in the search of this vessel, *trigonum Callo*. Its borders are the following: on the right is *ductus cysticus*, on the left is *ductus hepaticus communis*, from above is *a. cystica*. Practically for bandaging of vessels, surgeon searches a fork, which is formed by the *ductus cystous* and *ductus hepaticus communis*, from here goes up, where this vessel is located. A venous outflow from a gall-bladder is carried out to the system of janitrix, *v. portae*. Sphincter of Oddi is located in intraparietal part of bilious channel; it is a formation from the musculature of bilious motions. Sphincter of Westphal

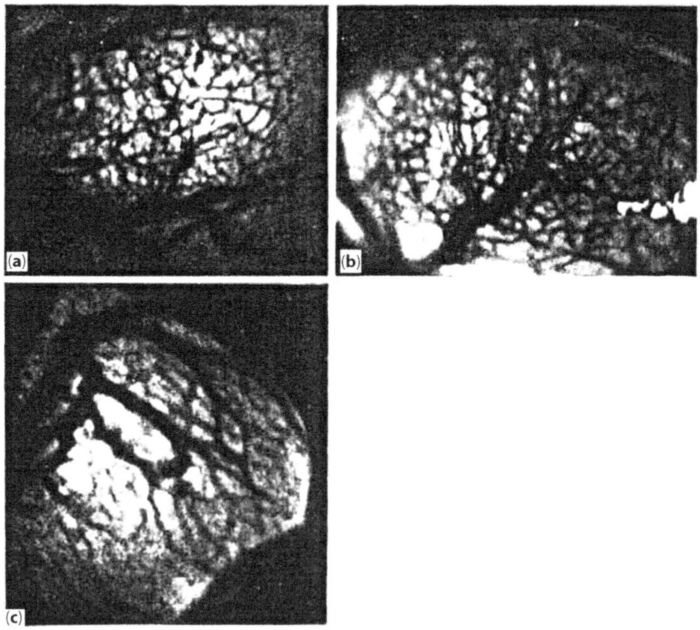

Figure 67 Non contrastive transillumination angiogram gallbladder.
a - major branches of the cystic artery in the fibrous layer; **b** - two veins that accompany cystic artery; c - “cell” of the bladder wall formed vessels.

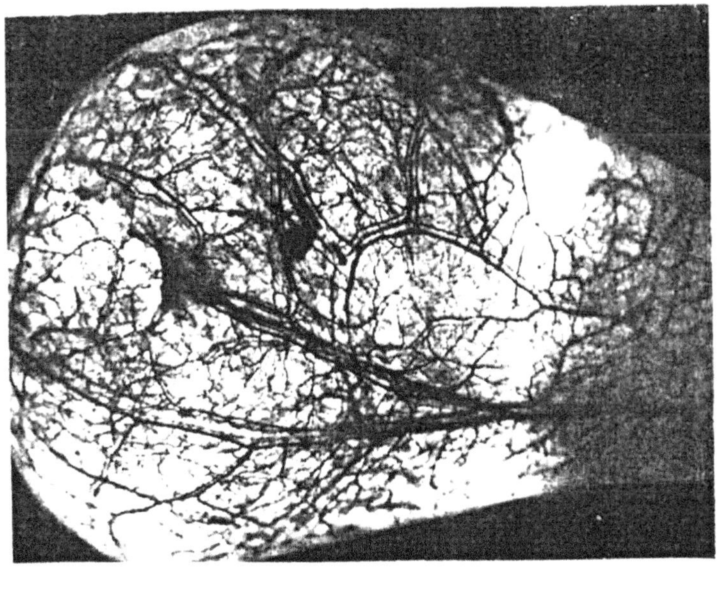

Figure 68 Transillumination pigment angiogram distal gallbladder.

The special expansion appears *diverticulum duodenale*, when it is connected with a Wirsung channel, mixing bile with pancreatic juice.

The spirally going valve appears in the area of gall-bladder neck, and also within the limits of *ductus cysticus.* It is called *valvula spiralis.*

The bile ductus have four sphincteres. They are under the influence of vegetative innervation, regulate the bile secretion into the gall-bladder or duodenum by eduction or weakening. Sphincter of Mirizzi is located under the place of confluence of the right and left bilious channels. Sphincter of Lyutkensa is located below than the place of confluence of *ductus hepaticus communis* and *ductus cysticus pancreaticus.* A vesico-colonic copula is presented on Figure 71.

Spleen, *lien, splen* is an essential organ in pathology. It carries many functions. The spleen has a scaphoid form. It has an external, protuberant diaphragmatic surface (*facies diaphragmatica*) and internal, concave medial surface (*facies medialis*) and also two ends: upper and lower (*extremitas superior et extremitas inferior*), and two sides: front and back. The internal surface of the spleen is subdivided into two fields. They are: front, whihc is called a gastric surface (*faces gastrica*), and back, which is a kidney surface (*facies renalis*).

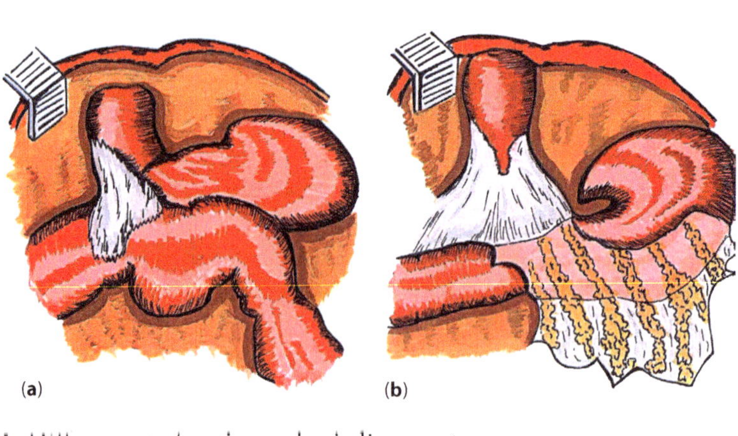

(a) (b)

Figure 71 Differences of vesico-colonic ligament.
a - on the one hand; 6 - the two sides of the bladder.

There is a small deepening on a medial surface of the lower pole of the kidney. It depends on fitting to transversal-rim bowel (*facies colica*). The spleen is an intraperitoneal organ. The peritoneum covers the spleen in three places. It is in the area of gate, and also at two its ends. It passes to other organs with formation of peritoneal copulas of spleen near two ends of the spleen.

Skeletopy of the spleen is determined in relation to ribs. It is located parallell to the ribs by its length. It lies between IX and XI ribs.

Projection of the spleen on a front and back wall of thoracal and abdominal cavities is important at any decision or question about the damage of one or other organs in spleen injury. The spleen is located close to the surface of the body by its posterior surface. It is projected on a shoulder-blade line. It does not come to the *linea paravertebralis* medially.

The chopped wound of the middle of one-third results in dissection of pleura cavity, without lung damage, because an injuring object goes into *sinus phrenicocostalis*. In spleen injury, in the area of its lower projection area, only a diaphragm is damaged, without dissection of pleura cavity. *Sinus phrenicocostalis* is partly filled by the lower edge of lung in breathing in.

In abdominal cavity injury at the front wall, at the level of the left costal arch on linea medioclavicularis a stomach is usually damaged, and a spleen adherent to it. It should be remembered that in breathing in the lower edge of lung covers the upper two-thirds of the spleen behind the diaphragm.

Syntopy. The spleen relates to the stomach, left kidney, transversal-rim bowel, to the tail of pancreas and to the diaphragm. *Facies diaphragmatica* is the largest surface of the spleen. *Facies gastrica* is a gastric surface of the spleen. It always adjoins the bottom of the stomach, without depending on the degree of stomach filling. *Facies renalis* is a kidney surface of the spleen. It adjoins the front surface and outward edge of the left kidney. *Facies colica* is a rim surface. It adjoins the transversal-rim bowel closely to the *flexura coli sinistra*. *Porta lienis* is a gate of the spleen. It adjoins the tail of pancreas on the lower part. There is a high, lower and medial location of the spleen.

Blood supply A. et v. lienalis.

Innervation. Left knots of sunny interlacement, left adrenal diaphragmatic interlacements.

Abnomalities of developments are lobular spleen, doubling of spleen, additional small spleens, confluence of spleen with a liver is rare.

The spleen of a newborn has a lobular structure. It is smoothed out gradually with age. Location of spleen can be high, when its upper edge is located at the level of VII rib. Location of the spleen can also be lower, when its upper edge corresponds to IX rib.

A pancreas (Figure 72) is subdivided into three parts: head, *caput pancreatis*, body, *corpus pancreatis*, and tail, *cauda pancreatis*.

The pancreas is situated behind the stomach, crosses a backbone in transversal direction, and lies extraperitoneally. Its head lies in the loops of the duodenum. The body lies on the backbone. Its tail reaches the spleen on the left. The ligamentous apparatus of the pancreas is presented by three copulas. They are gastrointestinal, pancreatic, pyloric, pancreatic and pancreatic-selelezenochnoy copulas.

Syntopy. At the front is a back wall of stomach, lower surface of liver, root of mesentery of transversal-rim bowel, loop of thin bowel; behind is *a v.porta, v. cava inferior*, aorta; above is a splenic artery and vein; below is a *a. et v. mesenterica superioris*; on the left is a gate of the spleen; on the right is a duodenum.

Projection. On a horizontal line, connecting the ends of 7th ribs on the right and on the left.

A blood supply is carried out by the system of celiac artery: *a. coeliaca, a. mesenterica superior, a. gastroduodenalis, rami pancreatici a. lienalis.*

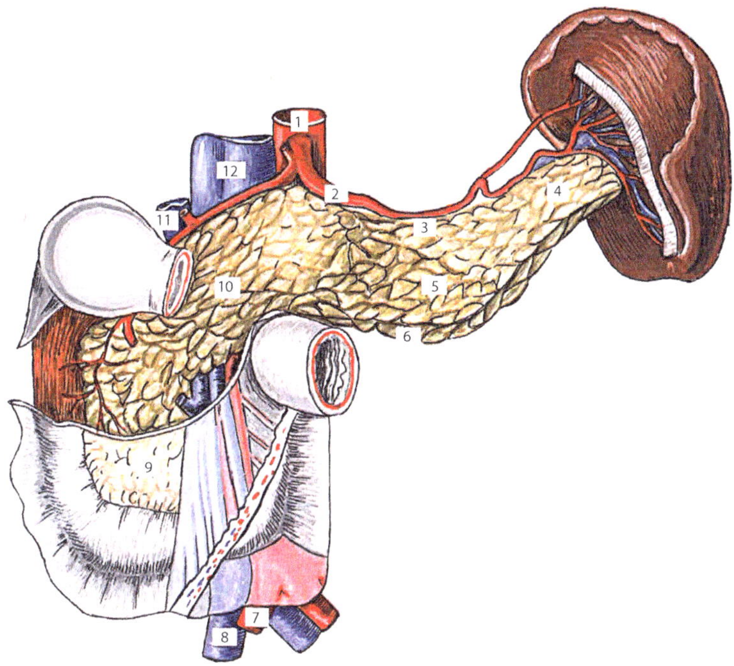

Figure 72 Pancreas.
1 – aorta; 2 – a. lienalis; 3 – margo superior; 4 – cauda pancreatis; 5 - margo anterior; 6 - margo inferior; 7 – a. iliaca communis; 8 – v. iliaca communis; 9 – caput pancreatic; 10 - corpus pancreatic; 11 – v. portae; 12 – v. cava inferior.

Innervation. *Plexus solaris* is a sunny interlacement; *plexus hepaticus anterior* is a front hepatic interlacement; *plexus hepaticus posterior* is a back hepatic interlacement; *plexus lienalis* is a splenic interlacement; *plexus mesentericus superior* is an upper mesenteric interlacement; *plexus renalis sinister* is the left kidney interlacement. All indicated interlacements accompany corresponding arterial trunks.

Abnomalities of development are trihedral form of gland, flat pancreas, angulate pancreas, lanceolate pancreas, s-shaped pancreas, circinate pancreas, tailed pancreas.

In the newborn, the pseudoagus gland is small (5–6 cm long, three times as large as at 10 years old), located deeply in the abdominal cavity, at the level of the X thoracic vertebra, in subsequent age periods - at the level of the I lumbar vertebra.

intermediate line, *sulcus intermedius*, between aponeurotic and muscular parts of *m. latissimi dorsi.*

Projection of organs on the skin of lumbar area. A “back kidney point”, i.e., the projection of kidney gate on a posterior abdominal wall, is determined in a corner between the lateral edge of the extensor of the back and the XI rib. The XII rib crosses the left kidney behind in the middle of it, the right kidney – between the upper and middle of one-thirds. The projection of pelves, as well as the beginning of ureters, corresponds to the projection of the kidney gate. Ureters are projected lower (from II - III of lumbar vertebrae), and their passage corresponds approximately to the vertical line, which goes on the outer ends of transverse processes of lumbar vertebrae. Adrenals are projected on the ends of transverse processes at the level of the XI intercostal space and the beginning of the XII rib. The projection of knots of the celiac plexus is determined on an area between two horizontal lines: the first one passes a bit higher than the inferior edge of the XII pectoral vertebra, the second one passes on the inferior edge of the I lumbar vertebra. An abdominal aorta is projected to the surfaces of bodies of XII thoracic and first 4 lumbar vertebrae, a few to the left of midline. Vena cava inferior is projected to the surfaces of bodies of 4 upper lumbar vertebrae, a few to the right of midline.

Age distinctions. Lumbar area in children under 3 years old is flat with the smoothed-out relief, which is explained by the weak expression of the bending of the backbone and the weak development of muscles. Intraperitoneal fascia, which forms the posterior wall of retroperitoneum, is very thin, tender and poorly expressed. Extraperitoneal fascia of newborns is presented by a thin semilucent plate, which sheets at the concave edge of the kidney are loose and break easily.

Paravertebral line, *linea paravertebralis*, i.e., a line conducted to the outer edge of the muscle and straightening the backbone, *m. erector spinae*, divides the lumbus on the lateral lumbar area, *regio lumbalis lateralis*, and the medial lumbar area, *regio lumbalis medialis*.

Layer topography of the outer (lateral) lumbar area (Figure 73):

1. Skin, *cutis*;
2. Depot fat, *panniculus adiposus*. The thickness of hypoderm of lumbar area is distributed evenly;

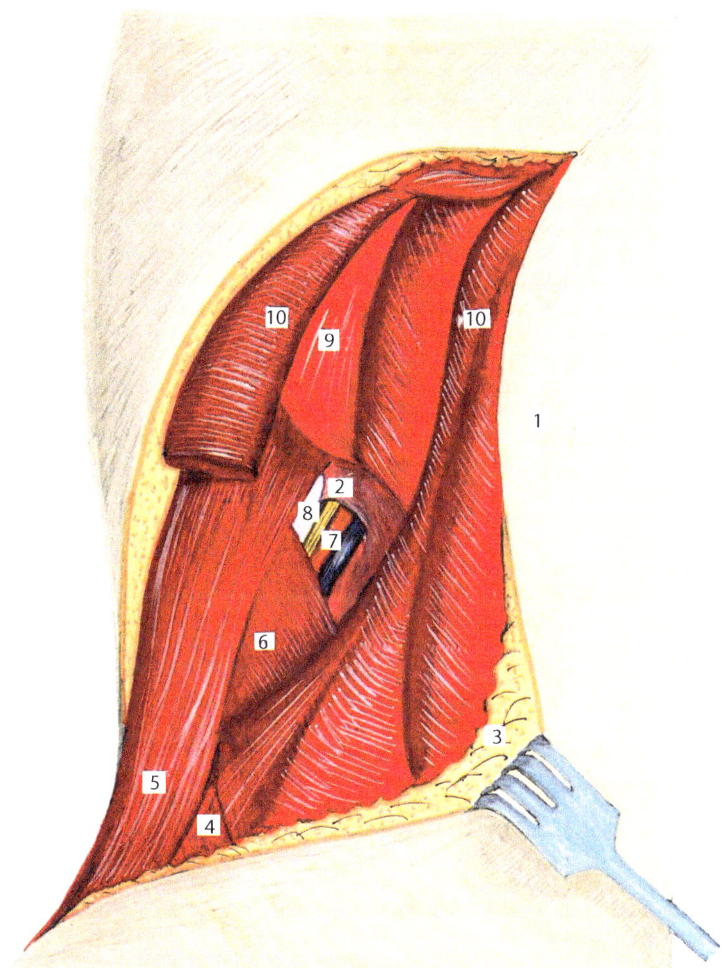

Figure 73 Lumbar region.
1 - derma; 2 - aponeurosis m.rectus abdominis; 3 - paniculus addiposus; 4 - triangle of Pte; 5 - m.obliquus externus abdominis; 6 - m.obliquus internus abdominis; 7 - subcostal vessels; 8 - costa (XII); 9 - m. serratus posterior inferior; 10 - m. latissimus dorsi.

3. Superficial fascia, *fascia superficialis*;

4. The fatty lumbar-gluteal mass, *massa adiposa lumboglutealis*, lies as a wide layer within the limits of lumbar area with passing to the gluteal area;

5. Lumbar-pectoral fascia, *fascia thoracolumbalis*, forms sheathes for muscles located in the examined area;

6. A latissimus, *m. latissimus dorsi*, goes from spinous processes of 6 lower pectoral and lumbar vertebrae, from the posterior surface of the sacrum and fourth of iliac crest and attaches to the crest of lesser tubercle of humeral bone;

7. The abdominal external oblique muscle, *m. obliquus abdominis externus*, attaches to the iliac crest throughout the front two-thirds, as a result between the external oblique muscle, the latissimus and the iliac crest the lumbar triangle (triangle of Pte, *trigonum lumbale*) appears, which is a weak place, a place of the exit of hernia, abscesses from retroperitoneal space.

8. The abdominal internal oblique muscle, *m. obliquus abdominis internus*, covers only the outside part of the studied area. In this way on the internal-upper part of the area there is a region without an internal oblique muscle. It is a lumbar quadrangle (quadrangle of Lesgaft-Grunfeld, *tetragonum lumbale*), where a pus can break through from a retroperitoneum. Its borders: upper is a posterior inferior serratus muscle, *m.serratus posterior inferior*, lower is an abdominal internal oblique muscle, *m. obliquus abdominis internus*, from within is a muscle straightening a backbone, *m. erector spinae*, outside is the XII rib.

9. Aponeurosis of the abdominal transversal muscle, *aponeurosis m. transversi abdominis*, is the bottom of the quadrangle;

10. The square muscle of lumbar, *m. quadratus lumborum*, with its lateral part lies in the medial part of the studied area;

11. Square fascia, *fascia quadrata*, is part of intraperitoneal fascia, *fascia endoabdominalis*, which lies on the square muscle of lumbar. Inwards there is an abdominal retroperitoneal space, *spatium retroperitoneale*.

Layered topography of the inner (medial) lumbar area:

1. The skin, *cutis*;

2. Depot fat, *panniculus adiposus*;

3. Superficial fascia, *fascia superficialis*;

4. Aponeurosis of latissimus dorsi, *aponeurosus m. latissimi dorsi*;

5. The superficial plate of lumbar-pectoral fascia, *lamina superficialis fasciae thoracolumbalis*, goes from the spinous processes of lumbar vertebrae;

6. Muscle, straightening the backbone, *m. erector spinae*, is located between the spinous and transversal processes of vertebrae.

7. The deep plate of lumbar-pectoral fascia, *lamina profunda fasciae thoracolumbalis*, goes from the transversal processes of lumbar vertebrae, overcoming a muscle straightening the backbone, *m. erector spinae*, at the front, unites with the superficial plate of the same fascia, passes to the aponeurosis of the abdominal transversal muscle, *aponeurosis m. transversi abdominis*. The area of the lumbar-pectoral fascia and aponeurosis of the abdominal transversal muscle between the XII rib and transversal processes of XI - XII thoracal and I lumbar

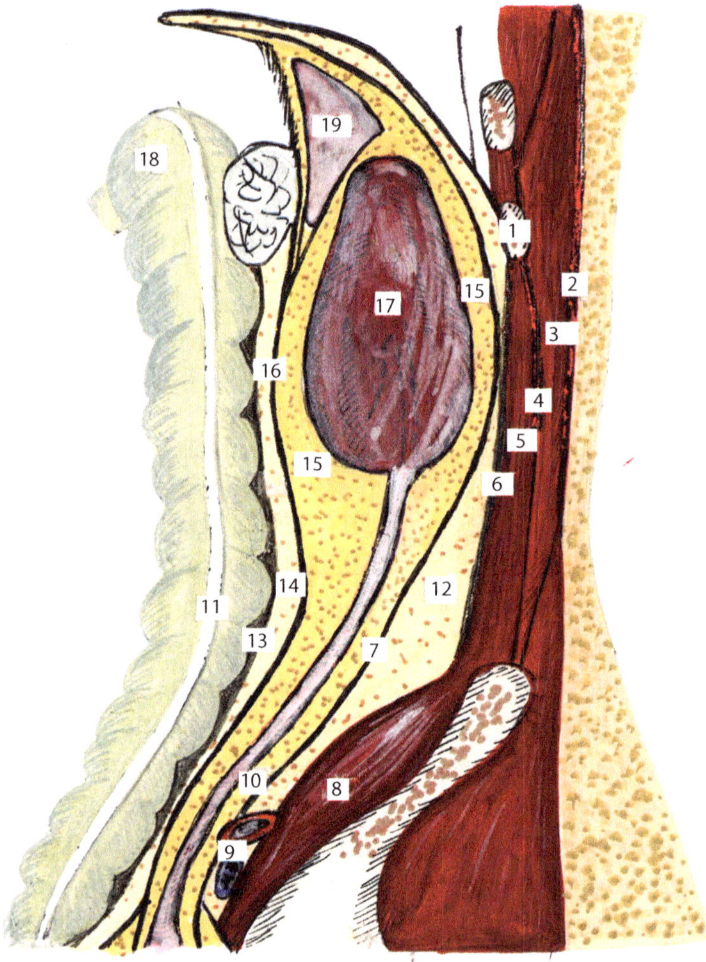

Figure 74 Topography of retroperitoneal space.
1 – costa; 2 – m. erector spinae; 3 – m. erector spinae; 4 – lamina profunda f. thoraco lumbalis; 5 – m. qudratus lumborum; 6 – fascia endoabdominalis; 7 – fascia intrarenalis; 8 – m. iliacus; 9 – common iliac vessels; 10 – ureter; 11 – taenia libera coli; 12 – retroperitoneal cellular layer; 13 – Told's fascia; 14 – retrocolon ligament; 15 – paniculus pararenalis; 16 – fascia prerenalis; 17- ren; 18 – intestinum crassum; 19 - suprarenalis

4. Renal adipose capsule (paranephric cellulose), *capsula adiposa renis*, is a loose fatty cellulose, which embraces a kidney from every side;

5. Kidney, *ren*, is covered by a dense fibrotic capsule, *capsula fibrosa renis*;

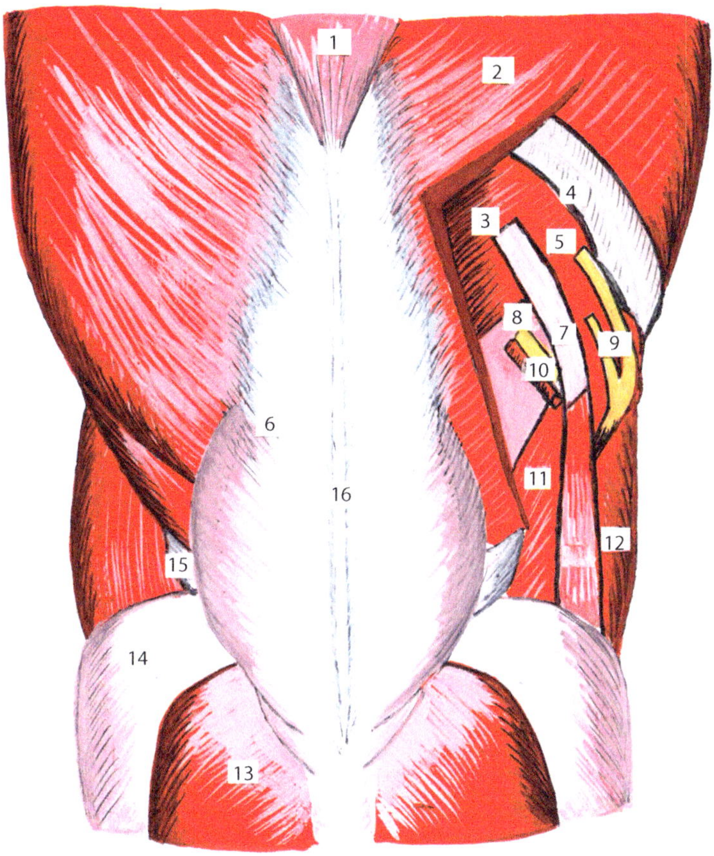

Figure 75 The posterior wall of the abdomen.
1 – m. trapezium; 2 – m. latissimus dorsi; 3 – m. serratus posterior inferior; 4 – costa (XI); 5 – mm. intracostales; 6 – fascia thoracolumbalis;7 – costa (XII); 8 – aponeurosis m. transversus abdominis; 9 – n. intercostalis (XI); 10 – subcostal vessels and nerves; 11 – m. obliquus internus abdominis; 12 – m. obliquus extemus abdominis; 13 – m. gluteus maximus; 14 – m. gluteus medius;15 – triangle of Pte; 16 – spinous processes of the lumbar vertebrae

6. Renal adipose capsule, *capsula adiposa renis (paranephron)*;
7. Prenephric fascia, *fascia prerenalis*, is the front sheet of the kidney fascia, *fascia renalis*, above and from sides it meets with retronephric fascia, below it passes to preureteric fascia, *fascia praeuteterica*. Prenephric and retronephric fasciae form a fascial bag for a kidney and its adipose capsule;

8. A paracolic cellulose, *paracolon*, is situated behind the ascending and descending colons. Above it achieves the mesenteric root of the transverse colon, below it arrives at the level of the blind gut on the right and the root of meso-sigmoid on the left, outside it is limited to attaching of the fascia renalis to the peritoneum, medially it comes to the root of mesostenium, behind it is limited to the prenephric and preureteric fasciae, at the front – to the peritoneum of lateral channels and retrocolic fascia.

9. Retrocolic fascia, Told's fascia, *fascia retrocolica,* appears at antenatal development as a result of the concretion of the sheet of a primary mesocolon with the parietal sheet, in a shape of a thin plate it lies between a cellulose, *paracolon*, and ascending or descending colon;

10. Colon, *colo*n: in a right lumbar area is an ascending colon, *colon ascendens*, in left – descending, *colon descendens*;

11. Visceral peritoneum, *peritoneum viscerale.*

Organs of Retroperitoneal Space (Figure 76)

Kidney (**Figure** 77), *ren, nephros*, is a pair organ, having the size of about 10x5x4 cm and mass of approximately 150 g, located in the upper department of the retroperitoneum. In every kidney it is accepted to distinguish anterior and posterior surfaces, lateral and medial edge, superior and inferior poles. In relation to the backbone the left kidney is situated at the level of Th11 - L2, and the gate - below the XII rib, a right kidney is situated at the level of Th12 - L2, the gate - at the level of the XII rib. On the concave medial edge of this organ there is a deepening – so-called kidney gate, from which a kidney hilum goes out.

The elements of kidney hilum are situated in the direction from front to back in a next sequence: kidney vein, kidney artery, pelvis. The branching of kidney artery is the basis for allocating of kidney segments. A kidney consists of 5 segments: 2 pole, 2 front and back. Kidneys are covered with the peritoneum extraperitoneally.

Syntopy of kidneys. Behind, the kidney adjoins closely to the lumbar part of the diaphragm, to the square lumbar muscle, to the transversal abdominal muscle, to the large lumbar muscle. Adrenals fit closely to the upper pole of kidneys. Right hepatic lobe, the descending part of

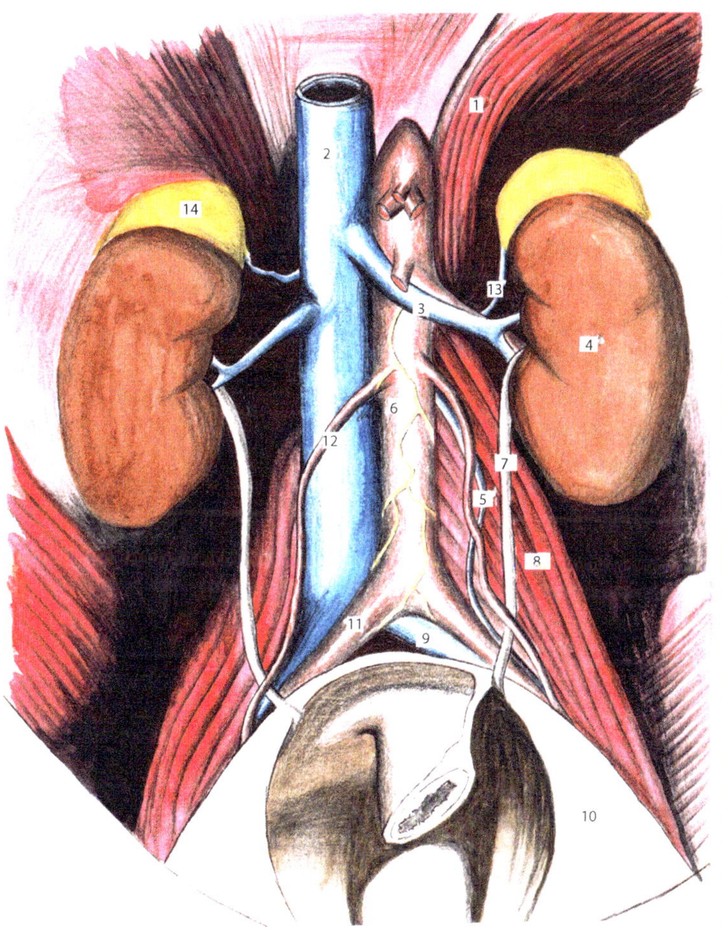

Figure 76 The organs and major blood vessels of the retroperitoneal space.
1 – diaphragma; 2 – v. cava inferior; 3 – v. renalis; 4 – ren; 5 – v. spermatica interim sinistra; 6 – aorta; 7 – ureter; 8 – m. lumbalis magna; 9 – v. iliaca communis sinistra; 10 – peritoneum parietale; 11 – a. iliaca communis dextra; 12 – v. spermatica; interna sinistra; 13 – v. suprarenalis; 14 – suprarenalis dexter

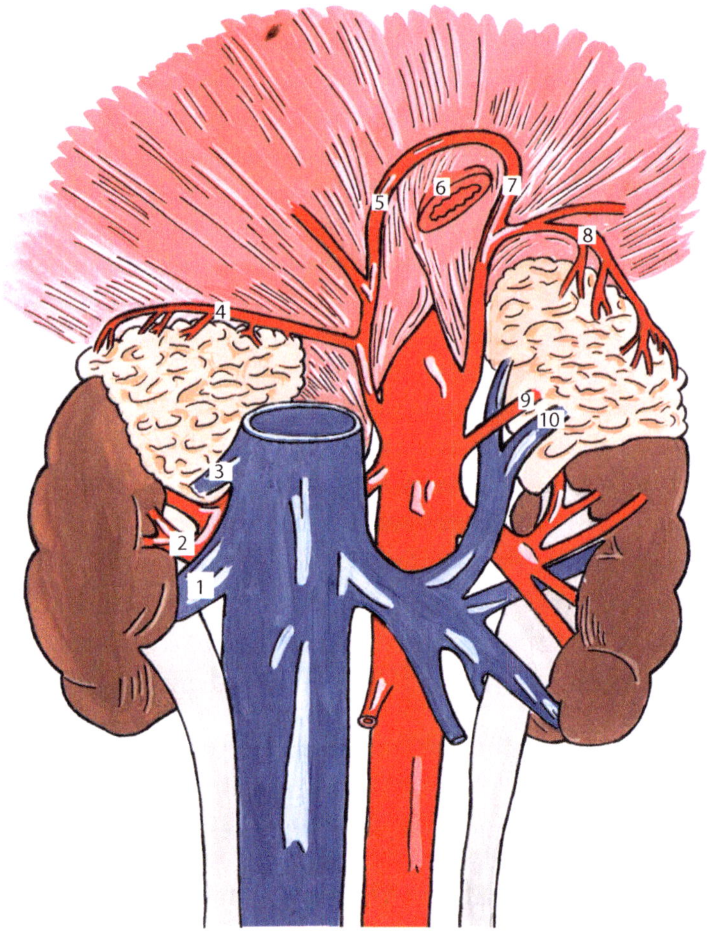

Figure 78 The blood vessels of kidneys and adrenal glands.
1 - v. renalis dextra; 2 - a. renalis dextra; 3 - v. suprarenalis dextra; 4 - a. suprarenalis superior dextra; 5 - a. phrenica inferior dextra; 6 - oesophagus; 7 - a. phrenica inferior sinistra; 8 - a. suprarenalis superior; 9 - a. suprarenalis media sinistra; 10 - a. suprarenalis sinistra

carried out with the same-name veins, flowing into the renal veins. Lymph flows away to the paraaortic lymphatic nodes.

The ureter, *ureter*, is a paired organ, which performs the secondary urine excretion from the kidney and connects the renal pelvis with the urinary bladder, it has a shape of a tube with the length of 30-35 cm and a diameter of 5-10 mm. The ureter is divided into the abdominal

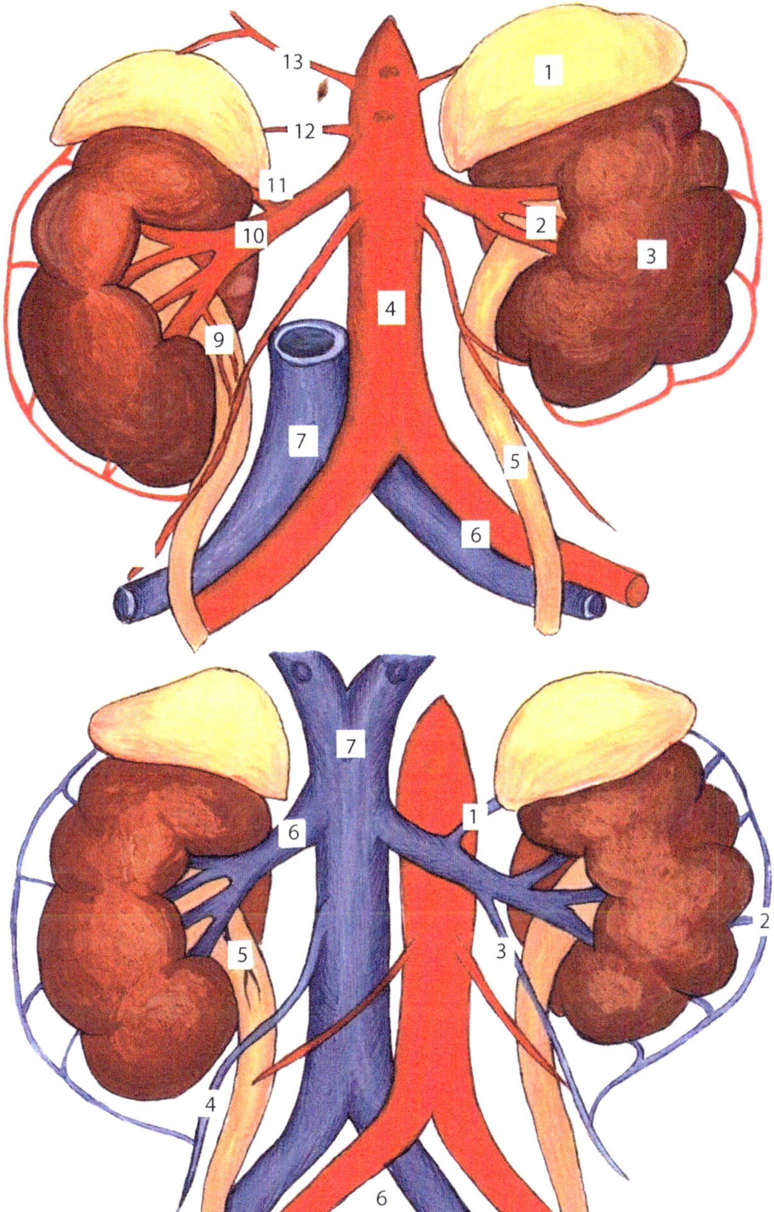

Figure 79 Kidney Vessels.
A — renal arteries: 1 - gl. Suprarenalis; 2 -hilus renalis; 3 - ren; 4 - pars abdominalis aortae; 5 - ureter; 6 - vasa iliaca communa; 7 - v. cava inferior; 8 - a. ovarica (testicularis); 9 - r. uretericus; 10 -a. renalis; 11 - a. suprarenalis inferoir; 12 - a. suprarenalis media; 13 - a. phrenica inferior;
B – renal veins: 1 -a. suprarenalis sinistra; 2 - plexus pampiniformis; 3 - a. ovarica (testicularis) sinistra; 4 - a. ovarica (testicularis) dextra; 5 - r. uretericus; 6 - v. renalis; 7 - v. cava inferior

portion, *pars abdominalis*, which goes from the renal pelvis to the border line, *linea terminalis*, and the pelvic portion, *pars pelvina*, which is located in the small pelvis. Throughout the ureter there are three narrowings: when passing from the kidney pelvis into the ureter, near the terminal line, and before flowing into the urinary bladder. Surrounded with the cellulose and the pre- and retro-ureteral fasciae, *fasciae praeureterica et retroureterici*, the ureters go down the large lumbar muscle, *m. psoas major*, together with the genitofemoral nerve, *n. genitofemoralis*, and near the terminal line bend over the external iliac artery on the right and over the common iliac artery on the left, going into the cellular spaces of the pelvis.

Syntopy (Figure 80). The following organs adjoin the right ureter: the duodenum, the parietal peritoneum of the right mesenteric sinus and the right colon vessels, *a. et v. colica dextra*, the root of the mesentery and the iliac colon vessels, *a. et v. ileocolica*, testicular (ovarian) vessels, *vasa testicularia (ovarica)* at the front; the ascending colon laterally; the inferior vena cava medially. The organs adjoin to the left ureter are the parietal peritoneum of the left mesenteric sinus and the left colonic vessels, *a. et v. colica sinistra*, the root of the mesentery of the sigmoid colon, sigmoid and upper rectal vessels, *a. et v. sigmoidea et rectalis superior*, testicular (ovarian) vessels at the front; the descending colon laterally; the aorta medially.

The blood supply is carried out with *aa. renalis, testicularis (ovarica) - pars abdominalis; a. rectalis media, vesicularis inferior - pars pelvina.* **Blood outflows** away with the *vv. testiculares (ovarisae), iliaca interna.* **Innervation**: *pars abdominalis - plexus renalis; pars pelvina - plexus hypogastricus.* **Lymph outflows**: from *pars abdominalis* - to *nodi lymphatici aortales abdominales*; from *pars pelvina* - to *nodi lymphatici iliaci.*

Features of sizes, shape and position of the organs of the retroperitoneal space in children (Figure 81). In newborns the kidneys are relatively large and have a lobed structure. The left kidney is usually slightly larger than the right. The average weight of the kidney is 12g. Both surfaces of the kidney (anterior and posterior) are bulging and

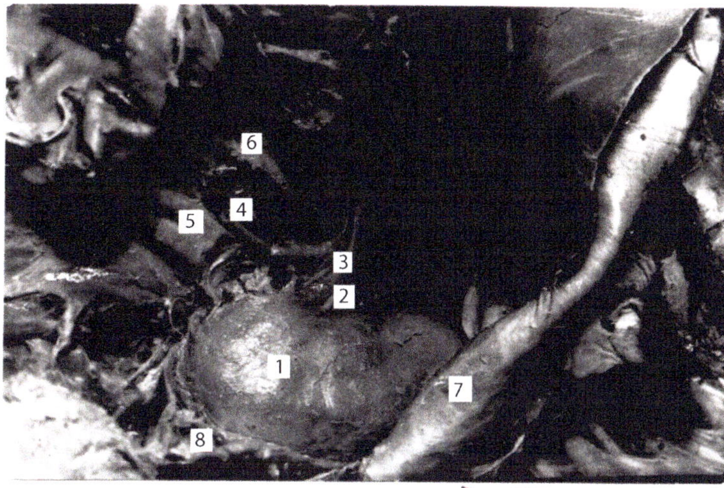

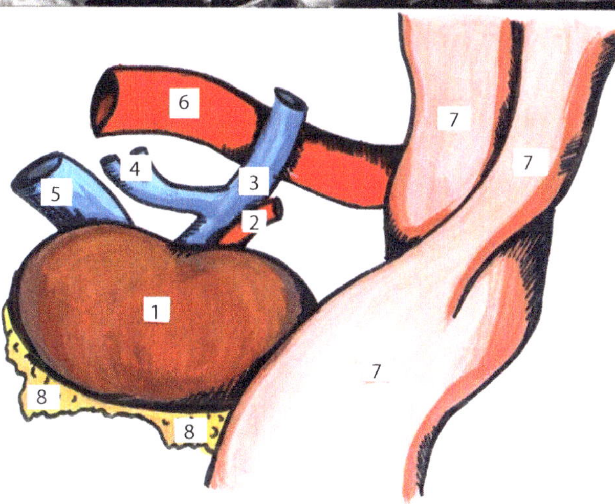

Figure 80 Kidney topography.
1 -ren; 2 - a. renalis dextra; 3 - v. renalis dextra; 4 - vv. lumbales; 5 - v. cava inferior; 6 - aorta abdominalis; 7 - peritoneum; 8 - capsula adiposa

rough. Sulci, separating the renal lobes, are visible on them. The outer edge is convex, the internal one is concave. The central part of the inner edge corresponds to the kidney gate. The major part of the renal pelvis is located extrarenally. The longitudinal axes of the kidneys are parallel to the spine or even have a divergent direction. The upper end of the left kidney is located at the level of the XII thoracic vertebra, the lower end is located at the level of the IV lumbar vertebra, the XII

the left one has a quadrangular shape up to 7 years old, and then the crescent shape. In newborns adrenal arteries are relatively short and have a straight course.

Surgical Anatomy of Congenital Malformations

The congenital displacement of the kidney, *dystopia renis congnita*, refers to its location below the normal level. In these cases, the renal artery begins from the vessels located at the same level. There are the following types of renal dystopias:

1. Iliac dystopia of the kidney, *dystopia renis iliaca*: usually in this case the kidney is in the iliac pit; the renal artery departs from either the distal aorta or from one of the iliac arteries;

2. Pelvic kidney dystopia, *dystopia renis pelvina*: the kidney occurs in the pelvis;

3. Abdominal dystopia, *dystopia renis abdominalis*: the kidney lies at the level of the lower lumbar vertebrae and, like the previous form, is firmly fixed by the vessels of this field.

   In relation to the midline of the body there are several variations of the pelvic dystopias:

   a. *dystopia renis monolateralis* - if the kidney is located on the side where it should be;

   b. *dystopia renis mediana* - if it is located in the midline of the body;

   c. *dystopia renis alterolateralls* - if the kidney is moved from its side to the opposite;

4. *Dystopia cruciata* - cross dystopia – if the location of the two kidneys on one side, one over another; ureters are crossed.

Horseshoe kidney. The horseshoe kidney with the junction of the lower poles, *ren arcuatus inferior.* If the metanephrogenic tissue of both sides is close to the spine and the lower poles of this tissue come in contact, then the horseshoe kidney with the lower neck develops. The horseshoe kidney with upper neck, *ren arcuatus superior.* Here the metanephrogenic tissue merges with its upper poles.

Narrowing (stricture) of the ureter is observed in 0.5-0.7% of children. The most common anomaly is localized in the vesicoureteral segment, then in the ureteropelvic segment, but can occur in any part of the ureter. The restriction can be unilateral or bilateral, single and multiple. Above the constriction of the ureter the pyelocaliceal system is expanded due to the continuous increase of pressure and the urine stagnation. If the obstruction is localized in the ureteropelvic junction, the hydronephrosis develops. When the location of the narrowing is in the prostatic part, in the middle third of the ureter it significantly expands and elongates above the obstruction level. The ureter becomes long, tortuous; its thickness can be equal to the colon.

The kidney duplication is accompanied by the ureter duplication. In most cases, both ureters open with two ureteral orifices into the urinary bladder, with the ureteral orifice of the upper pelvis falling into the bladder below the ureteral orifice of the lower pelvis or one of the ureteral orifices can be ectopic. Sometimes there is the union of the duplicated ureter in the pelvic part with one orifice in the bladder – split ureter.

Congenital hydronephrosis is an enlargement of the renal pelvis and calyces. It develops due to the difficulties of urine outflow as a result of: the ureteropelvic junction stenosis; the compression of the ureter by the extra renal artery, coming to the lower pole of the kidney; the inflection or compression of the ureter by the synechias; the presence of the valve, which is a plication of the mucous membrane of the ureter.

Vessels and nerves of the retroperitoneal space. The abdominal aorta *(pars abdominalis aortae)* lies on the anterior surface of the spine, to the left of the median sagittal plane, from XII thoracal to IV-V lumbar vertebrae, where it is divided into its terminal branches – the right and the left common iliac arteries, *aa. iliaca communis dextra et sinistra.* The common iliac artery from the aortic bifurcation goes to the sacroiliac joint, *articulatio sacroiliaca*, where it is divided into external and internal iliac arteries, *aa. iliaca externa et interna*. The organs adjoin to the abdominal aorta are the following: behind – the bodies of ThXII-LIV; at front – the parietal peritoneum of the posterior wall of omental bursa, the pancreas, the ascending part of the duodenum and the root of the mesentery; on the right – vena cava inferior; on the left – the left adrenal gland, the inner edge of the left kidney, lumbar nodes of the left sympathetic trunk. The following branches depart from the abdominal aorta:

Parietal: inferior diaphragmatic artery, a. *phrenica inferior*, pair, extends at the level of XII thoracic vertebra; lumbar arteries, *aa. lumbales*, 4 pair arteries, extend from the lateral surfaces of the aorta; median sacral artery, *a. sacralis mediana*, departs at the level of LV.

Visceral: celiac trunk, *truncus coeliacus*, departs at the level of ThXII, divides into splenic, common hepatic and left gastric arteries, *aa. lienalis, hepatica communis et gastrica sinistra*; middle suprarenal artery, *a. suprarenalis media*, pair, departs at the level of I lumbar vertebra; superior mesenteric artery, *a. mesenterica superior*, unpaired, departs slightly below the previous artery at the level of LI; renal artery, *a. renalis*, pair, departs at the level of LI- LII; testicular (ovary) artery, *a. testicularis (a. ovarica),* pair, extends from the front surface of the aorta at the level of LIII- LIV; inferior mesenteric artery, *a. mesenterica inferior*, unpaired, departs at the level of LIII.

The lower hollow vein, *v. cava inferior* is formed on the front surface of the spine to the right of the median sagittal line at the level of LIV-LV at the confluence of the common iliac veins, *vv. ilacae communes*, and leaves the abdominal cavity through the aperture of the same name. The organs adjoin to the vena cava inferior are: behind – the bodies of ThXII - LIV; at the front – the liver, the peritoneum, bounding the epiploic foramen behind, the head of the pancreas and the portal vein, the lower horizontal part of the duodenum, and the root of the mesentery; on the left – the abdominal aorta; on the right – the right adrenal gland, the inner edge of the right kidney, right ureter, lumbar nodes of the right sympathetic trunk. The next veins flow into the inferior vena cava: lumbar veins, *vv. lumbales* - 4 paired veins; the right testicular (ovarian) vein, *v. testicularis (ovarica) dextra*; the left testicular (ovarian) vein goes into the left renal vein, *v. renalis sinistra*; renal veins, *vv. Renales*, at the level of I-II of the lumbar vertebrae; the right adrenal vein, *v. suprarenalis*, goes into the left renal vein; hepatic veins, *vv. hepaticae*; lower diaphragmatic veins, *vv. phrenicae inferiores.*

The azygos, *v. azygos*, and **hemiazygos**, *v.hemiazygos* veins go up the anterolateral surfaces of the spine, being a continuation of the ascending lumbar veins, *vv. lumbales ascendens*. They are transformed into the corresponding veins of the chest cavity.

The thoracic duct behind the right edge of the abdominal aorta rises up and over the aortic aperture of the diaphragm, and enters the chest cavity, where it lies in the groove between the aorta and the azygos vein, v. *azygos*. The thoracic duct goes into the left subclavian vein, *v. subclavia*, near the jugular venous angle, *angulus venosus juguli*.

The lumbar plexus, *plexus lumbalis* – the upper part of the lumbosacral plexus. This plexus of somatic nerves is formed with the anterior branches of spinal nerves from segments ThXII - LIV. The branches of the plexus innervate the muscles of the abdominal wall and thigh, and provide the sensitivity of the parietal peritoneum and skin of the hypogastrium and thigh:

- **Iliohypogastric nerve**, *n. iliohypogastricus*, (ThXII -LI) comes from the lateral edge of the large lumbar muscle, runs along the front surface of the square loin muscle, the inner surface of the transverse muscle, pierces it and lies between the internal oblique and transverse muscles, providing the sensory and motor phases of the abdominal reflex. It has two branches. The lateral cutaneous branch,

coming to the celiac nodes are the following: the fibers in composition of the large visceral nerve, *n. splanchnicus major*, and partly the small visceral nerve, *n. splanchnicus minor*, fibers from the thoracic aortic plexus, fibers from the vagus nerves, *nn. vagi*, fibers from the right phrenic nerve, *n. phrenicus dexter*. The branches of the plexus after the furcation of the celiac trunk form the secondary plexuses: hepatic, *plexus hepaticus*, splenic, *plexus lienalis*, gastric, *plexus gastrici*, pancreatic, *plexus pancreaticus*, reaching the relevant organs by the vessels:

- **Superior mesenteric plexus**, *plexus mesentericus superius*, unpaired, is situated on the homonymous artery and its branches. Superior mesenteric node, *ganglion mesentericus superius*, is located at the beginning of the superior mesenteric artery. To the superior mesenteric plexus the fibers come from the large, small and the lowest visceral nerves, *n.splanchnicus major, minor et imus*, and the vagus nerves, *nn. vagi*;

- **Renal plexus**, *plexus renalis*, paired, accompanies the renal arteries, has aortorenal nodes, *ganglia aortorenalia*, lying on the lateral surface of the aorta, at the beginning of the renal artery, and renal nodes, *ganglia renalia*, lying on the renal artery. The fibers of the small and lowest visceral nerves, *nn. splanchnici minor et imus*, lumbar visceral nerves and vagus nerves, *nn. vagi*, come to the plexus.

- **Ureteral plexus**, *plexus uretericus*, in the upper parts is formed from the fibers of a renal plexus, in the lower – from the fibers of the pelvic visceral nerves and the branches of the lower hypogastric plexus;

- **Ovarian (testicular) plexus,** *plexus ovaricus (testicularis)*, is formed from fibers of the renal plexus, along the same-name vessels comes to the ovarium (testicle);

- **Intermesenteric plexus,** *plexus intermesentericus*, is located on the aorta between the mesenteric arteries;

- **Inferior mesenteric plexus,** *plexus mesentericus inferior*, is located on the same-name artery and its branches, has the inferior mesenteric node, *ganglion mesentericus inferior*, located on the aorta at the site of origin of the inferior mesenteric artery. To the inferior mesenteric plexus the fibers come from the small and the lowest visceral nerves and the lumbar visceral nerves. Along the branches of the inferior mesenteric artery they reach the descending colon, sigmoid colon, and the upper part of the rectum.

Lymphatic vessels and regional lymph nodes. The lumbar lymph nodes, *nodi lymphatici lumbales*, collect lymph from the posterior wall of the abdomen and the common iliac lymph nodes, *nodi lymphatici iliaci communes*, and are located in the retroperitoneal space along the abdominal aorta and inferior vena cava. There are several groups of lumbar lymph nodes:

- **Left lumbar lymph nodes**, *nodi lymphatici lumbales sinistri*: lateral aortic lymph nodes, *nodi lymphatici aortici laterales*; preaortic lymph nodes, *nodi lymphatici praeaortici*; postaortic lymph nodes, *nodi lymphatici postaortici*;

- **Right lumbar lymph nodes**, *nodi lymphatici lumbales dextri*: lateral caval lymph nodes, *nodi lymphatici cavales laterales*; precaval lymph nodes, *nodi lymphatici praecavales*; postcaval lymph nodes, *nodi lymphatici postcavales.*

The right and left lumbar lymph nodes give the origin to the right and left lumbar trunks, *truncus lumbalis dexter et sinister*. At the confluence of these trunks the thoracic duct, *ductus thoracicus*, is formed in the initial part of which there is an extension – chylocyst, *cisterna chili*.

Chylocyst has a length of 1–6 cm and a diameter of 1–2 cm, and is most often located at the level of L1- LII. It gets the lymph from the intestinal lymph trunks, celiac, *nodi lymphatici coeliaci*, and superior mesenteric, *nodi lymphatici mesenterici superiors*, lymph nodes.

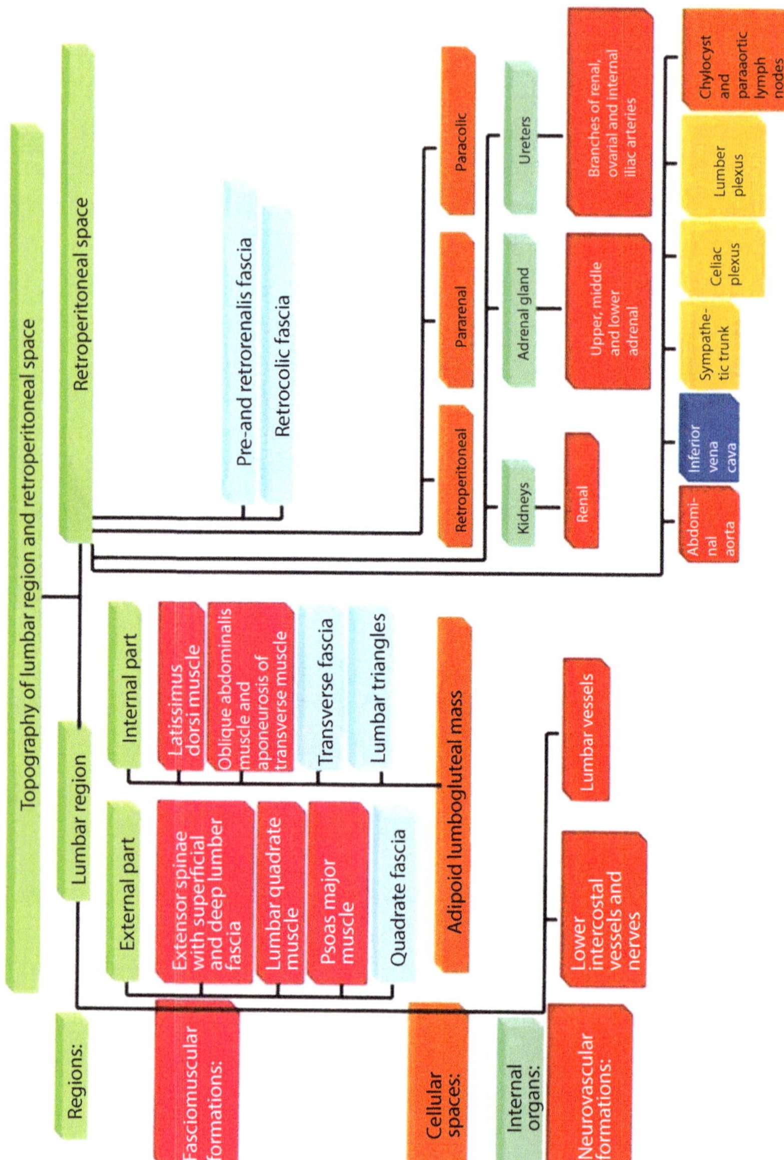
Topography of lumbar region and retroperitoneal space
Regions:
Lumbar region
Retroperitoneal space
Fasciomuscular formations:
External part
Extensor spinae with superficial and deep lumber fascia
Lumbar quadrate muscle
Psoas major muscle
Quadrate fascia
Internal part
Latissimus dorsi muscle
Oblique abdominalis muscle and aponeurosis of transverse muscle
Transverse fascia
Lumbar triangles
Pre-and retrorenalis fascia
Retrocolic fascia
Cellular spaces:
Adipoid lumbogluteal mass
Retroperitoneal
Pararenal
Paracolic
Internal organs:
Kidneys
Adrenal gland
Ureters
Neurovascular formations:
Lower intercostal vessels and nerves
Lumbar vessels
Renal
Upper, middle and lower adrenal
Branches of renal, ovarial and internal iliac arteries
Abdomi-nal aorta
Inferior vena cava
Sympathe-tic trunk
Celiac plexus
Lumber plexus
Chylocyst and paraaortic lymph nodes

Pathotography Chest

Fibroadenoma of mammary gland is a compaction in the chest, which often appears on one side of the upper part of the mammary gland. The tumor is elastic and smooth in palpation. In contrast to cancer, fibroadenoma is mobile because it is not attached to the skin. This benign formation can be of different sizes. More common are adenomas of small size about 3-8 millimeters in diameter. Rarely fibroadenoma grows up to 15 centimeters or grows on all the surface of the mammary gland. There may be a bulging of the subcutaneous "ball" or visual deformity of the breast, an increase of its size.

There are the following forms of fibroadenoma:

- immature form is characteristic of "juvenile fibroadenomas" that appears during teenage years and youth; a distinctive feature is the absence of an external capsule in a tumor;

a. endobronchial (exophytic and endophytic);

b. eribronchial (nodular and branched).

2. Peripheral cancer, which comes from the epithelium of subsegmental and smaller bronchi:

a. intra-branch node;

b. subpleural form, including cancer of Pankosta.

3. Bronchioloalveolar cancer, which comes from the epithelium of bronchioles and alveoli.

Pathotopogaphy (Figure 84). ***Central lung cancer*** occurs in 50% of cases. A tumor in the wall of the main, lobar or segmental bronchus causes its occlusion, which first leads to hypoventilation, and then to atelectasis of the ventilated area. In the exophytic form of the central cancer the tumor grows into the bronchus lumen; in the endophytic form it extends in the bronchus wall along the axis, deforming and narrowing its gap, subsequently leading to atelectasis.

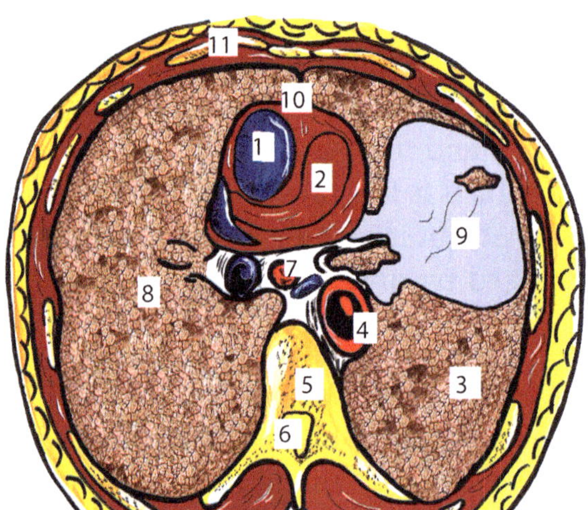

Figure 84 Transverse section of the chest.
1 – atrium dexter; 2 – ventriculus sinister; 3 – pulmo sinister; 4 – aorta descendens; 5 – columna vertrebralis; 6 – canalis spinalis; 7 – oesophagus; 8 - pulmo dexter; 9 – tumor node; 10 – facies cardiaca anterior; 11 – paries thoracica anterior

On x-ray atelectasis is characterized by a decrease in the volume ventilated by the affected area and a decrease in transparency or its complete airlessness with the presence of even, slightly concave contours. The peribronchial form of the central cancer doesn't appear in the initial stages as brightly as the endobronchial form because the violation of bronchial patency develops slowly. Peribronchially branched form of the central cancer is not accompanied by the formation of a tumor node, but grows as a diffuse infiltrate around the bronchus.

The feature of ***peripheral cancer*** is the long asymptomatic course of the disease because the tumor is located in the peripheral parts of the lung. The first signs of the disease are manifested only when the tumor grows and sprouts into the pleura, chest wall or bronchi of the 2-3rd order. X-ray sign of the peripheral tumor is a knot, usually round, with an uneven hummocky contour. The use of CT can most accurately identify the main radiographic signs of peripheral cancer.

A tumor can consist of several nodes, what is clearly visualized by CT. The structure of the tumor node may be heterogeneous due to the hypodense regions caused by decay or because of the presence of calcinates. The main characteristic CT signs are the radial contour of the tumor node, the tendon to the costal pleura, which is unevenly thickened at the lesion level and is often drawn into the node (a symptom of "umbiliculation"). On the MR-tomogram all the anatomical structures are visible as well as the skeletopy of the chest cavity organs: the thyroid gland is located 2 cm above the sternum, the heart is located at the level of the III-IV thoracic vertebrae, the liver is located at the level of V-XII right ribs. On the MR-tomogram of the patient with the revealed tumor node, it is possible to see violations of the integrity of the vertebra – the tumor sprouts its body, also shifts slightly downwards and the parenchyma of the lung.

Bronchioloalveolar cancer comes from the epithelium of bronchioles and alveoli and is characterized by a peculiar clinical and radiological manifestation. The tumor grows infiltratively and develops at the level of the alveoli and terminal bronchioles, necroses occur with tissue disintegration and the formation of microcavities. A very characteristic clinical sign is the presence of a large number of foamy phlegm in pink color. Cancer can also occur as a nodular and disseminated form. A distinctive feature in both cases is the heterogeneous ("cellular") structure of the tumor nodes.

Pulmonectomy is a surgical intervention that involves complete removal of the lung, which is performed due to pathological changes in the organ that threaten the life of the patient. Radical pulmonectomy involves the removal of the affected lung and regional lymph nodes, in which metastases are detected. Extended pulmonectomy is the removal of the lung and the anatomical structure, which is affected by metastases (for example, the pericardial flap or part of the diaphragm). The main radical operations for lung cancer are pneumonectomy and lobectomy and their variants (expanded or combined pneumonectomy, lobectomy with circular or sphenoid resection of the bronchi, bilobectomy, etc.).

Pathotopography (Figure 85). Especially interesting is the desolation of the cavity remaining after pneumonectomy. The dimensions of the cavity are different and depend on the growth, constitution and displacement of the mediastinum before the operation.

At the first time after surgery the pleural cavity remaining after lung removal is filled with air and partially exudate that consists of a tissue fluid with a certain admixture of blood. The cavity is emptied by the displacement of the mediastinum, an increase in the level of the diaphragm and the occlusion of the chest wall. Most of the cavity volume is reduced by increasing the dome of the diaphragm, less due to the mediastinum and even less due to the ribs. The dome of the diaphragm sometimes rises to the second rib (in front), and this process on the right side occurs somehow more slowly than on the left, which is probably due to the presence of such a massive organ as the liver. Different departments of the mediastinum are shifted in different ways. The lower and upper mediastinum are most mobile, the mediastinum middle in the region of the trachea bifurcation and the aortic arch is more firmly fixed to the spine. Not only the heart is displaced, but all other organs of the mediastinum: esophagus, trachea, large vessels including the

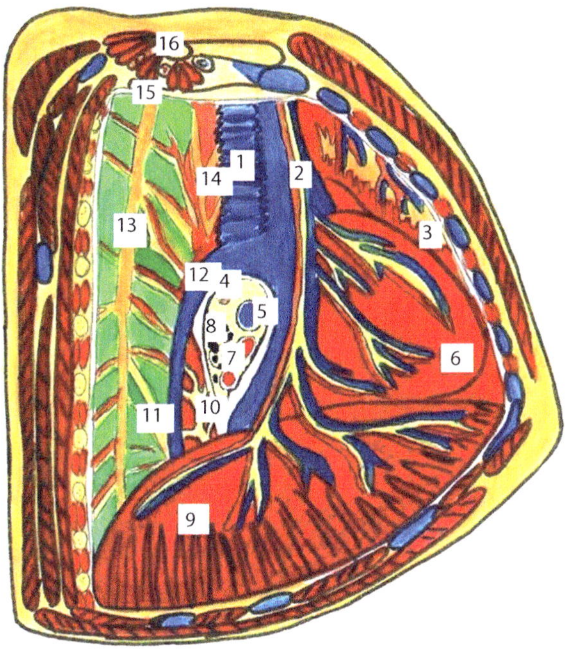

Figure 85 Mediastinum after removal of the right lung. Right view.
1 – trachea; 2 – n. phrenicus; 3 – thymus; 4 – bronchus principalis dexter; 5 – a. pulmonalis dexter; 6 – cor; 7 – vv. pulmonales dexter; 8 – nodi lymphatici bronchopulmonales; 9 – diaphragma; 10 – plexus esophagalis; 11 – n. splanchnicus major; 12 – v. azigos; 13 – truncus sympathicus; 14 – esophagus; 15 – costa; 16 – clavicular

thoracic aorta. After the completion of the moving processes in chest organs, a small space of the residual pleural cavity remains, which in most patients is filled with serous fluid. Sometimes there is a complete overgrowth of the cavity with connective tissue. All the above observations and data from special physiological studies show that people overcome well the removal of the lobe and the whole lung and in most cases they fully compensate for the functions of respiration and hemodynamics and consequently the restoration of work capacity.

Pneumonectomy (typical or radical) is performed in central carcinoma in case of lesion of the lobar bronchi with involvement of the main bronchus in the process, peripheral cancer with significant damage to the neighboring lobe, multiple metastases to the lymph nodes, several zones of regional metastasis and tumor infiltration of the vessels of the lung root, regardless of localization and growth pattern of

Vascular formations (angiomas) occur in benign liver tumors most often. They have a cavernous spongy structure and come from the venous network of the liver. Among the vascular tumors of the liver, there are cavernous hemangiomas and cavernomas. Nodular hyperplasia of the liver develops as a result of local circulatory and biliary disorders in certain zones of the liver. Macroscopically, this liver tumor can have a dark red or pink color, small-hulled surface, different size. The consistency of nodular hyperplasia of the liver is dense, the phenomena of local cirrhosis are microscopically detected. The degeneration of knotty hyperplasia in a malignant tumor of the liver is not excluded.

Pathotopography (Figures 87, 88). The danger of a hemangioma of the liver is a high probability of tumor rupture with the development of bleeding into the abdominal cavity and haemobilia (bleeding into the bile ducts), the torsion of the tumor's foot. In complicated cases, there may be a rupture of adenoma with the development of hemoperitoneum.

On the MR-tomogram, the syntopy of the abdominal cavity is visible: the rectus abdominis muscle, the left lobe of the liver to which the stomach adjoins from the left, the medial-inferior vena cava, delimited from the abdominal aorta by the diaphragm. The thoracic lymphatic duct is located on the right side of the abdominal aorta, which contacts the left lung, behind – the thoracic vertebra, containing the vertebral canal and the spinal cord.

On a computer tomogram, a diffuse-focal lesion of the liver parenchyma is seen in the form of rounded areas of darkening (neoplasm of unknown etiology). The liver is enlarged, pushing the stomach more laterally, the inferior vena cava is not visible. The left bend of the small intestine, unlike the normal picture, is not visible. All lobes of the liver and spleen are enlarged.

Hemangioma of the liver is a disease accompanied by the formation of a benign tumor. Very often, the hemangioma of the liver is a combination of vascular neoplasm of blastomatous and disembryoplastic character.

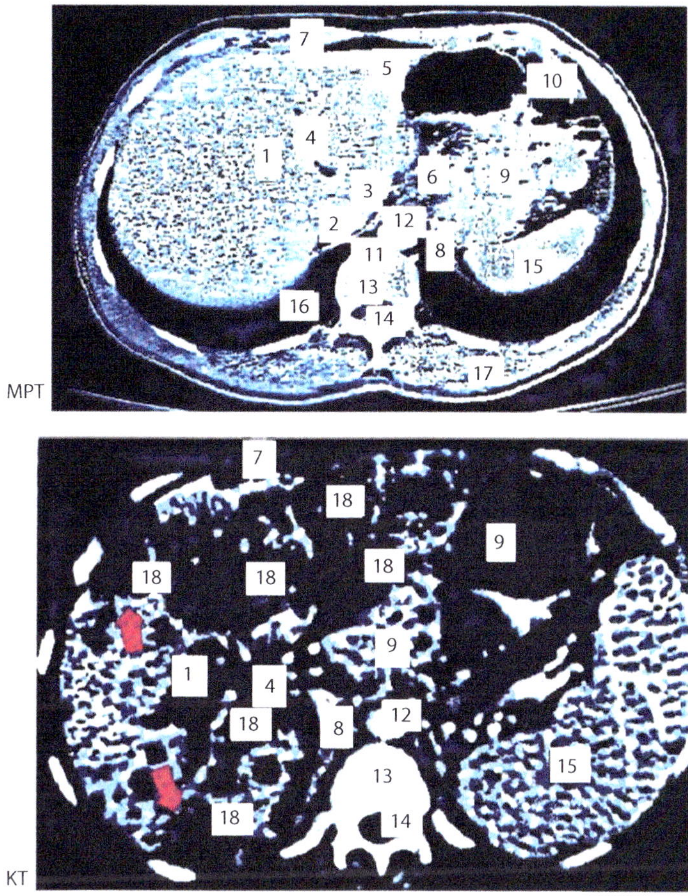

Figure 87 Cross section of the thorax at the level of the liver.
1,3,5 – lobes of the liver; 2 – inferior vena cava; 4 – a slot of a circular ligament and a circular ligament; 6 – lesser omentum; 7 – rectus abdominis muscle; 8 – diaphragm; 9 – stomach; 10 – left bend of the small intestine; 11 – thoracic lymphatic duct; 12 – abdominal aorta; 13 – thoracic spine; 14 – vertebral canal and spinal cord; 15 – the spleen; 16 – left lung; 17 – back muscles; 18 – neoplasm of the liver.

According to the structure and structure of education, hemangiomas are divided into two types:

1. Capillary - a benign tumor consisting of several separate small vascular cavities that are filled with blood. Usually each of these cavities feeds a separate blood vessel. Such growth can reach 2–3 cm in diameter.

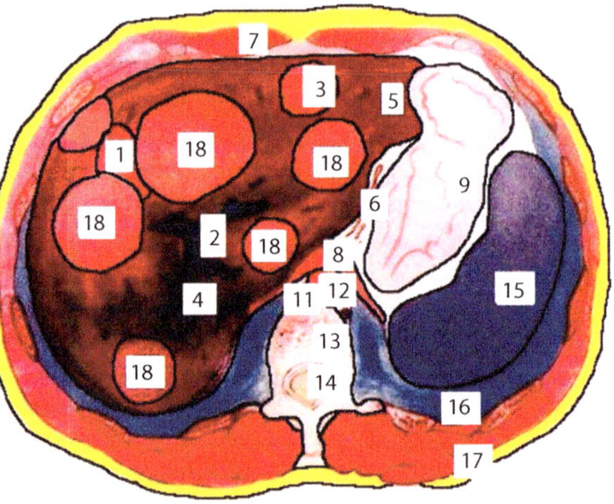

Figure 88 Cross section of the thorax at the level of the liver.
1 – lobulus hepatus dexter; 2 – v.cava inferior; 3 – lobulus hepatus caudatus; 4 – v.porta; 5 – lobus hepatus sinister; 6 – a.gastrica sinistra; 7 – m.rectus abdominis; 8-diafragma; 9 – gaster; 10 – flexura colica sinistra; 11 – nodus limfaticus thoracica; 12 – aorta abdominalis; 13 – vertebra thoracica; 14 – medulla spinalis et canalis vertebralis; 15 – spleen; 16 – pulmo dexter; 17 – m.latissimus dorsi; 18- neoplasm in the liver

2. Cavernous hemangioma of the liver - a benign tumor that is a few vascular cavities filled with blood and fenced off from each other by thin vascular walls. Such hemangioma can reach 20 cm in diameter and on a computer tomogram, a diffuse-focal lesion of the liver parenchyma is seen in the form of rounded areas of darkening (neoplasm of unknown etiology). The liver is enlarged, pushing the stomach more laterally, the inferior vena cava is not visible. The left bend of the small intestine, unlike the normal picture, is not visible. All lobes of the liver and spleen are enlarged.

Hemangioma of the liver is a disease accompanied by the formation of a benign tumor. Very often, the hemangioma of the liver is a combination of vascular neoplasm of blastomatous and disembryoplastic character.

According to the structure and structure of education, hemangiomas are divided into two types:

1. Capillary - a benign tumor consisting of several separate small vascular cavities that are filled with blood. Usually each of these cavities feeds a separate blood vessel. Such a growth can reach 2–3 cm in diameter.
2. Cavernous hemangioma of the liver - a benign tumor that is a few vascular cavities filled with blood and fenced off from each other by thin vascular walls. Such a hemangioma can reach 20 cm in diameter and occupy the whole right side of the liver. This is the most dangerous form, because excessive overflow of intracellular fluid or plasma can provoke rapid growth of the tumor.

Pathotopography (Figure 89). Hemangiomas of small size (up to 5.0 cm in diameter) do not appear clinically, however, for large (> 10 cm) and giant (> 15 cm) tumor sizes, pain syndrome, signs of compression

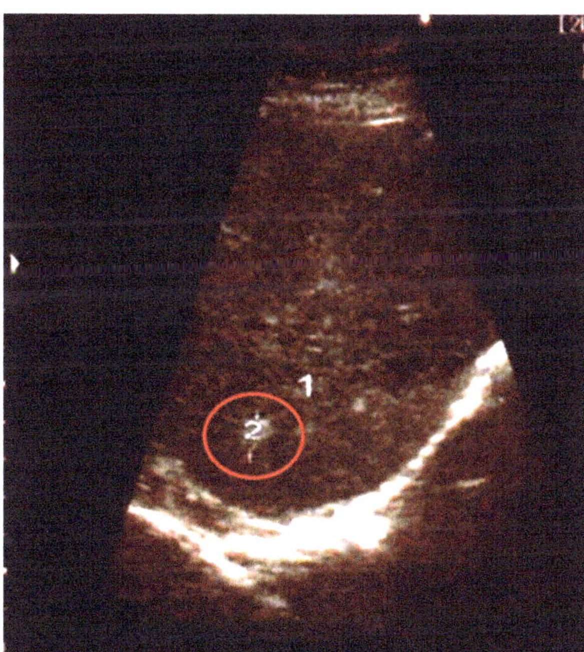

Figure 89 Hemangioma of the liver.
1 – right lobe of the liver; 2 – hemangioma of the right lobe of the liver

4. The symptom of the "target" is a decrease in the echostructure around the periphery of the focus and its amplification in the center (malignant liver tumor).

Thus, the information content of ultrasound examination of the liver is quite high, especially with focal lesions of the organ.

The additional lobe of the spleen is part of the splenic tissue of small size, located separately from the spleen itself. The main reason for the formation of an additional lobe is the developmental dysfunction at certain points in the intrauterine development of the child. This spleen can be very small, and can grow to a fairly large size. As a rule, they are covered with a peritoneum. This is very important to remember, because when there are indications for splenectomy (except for cases of traumatic rupture, tumors and cysts of the spleen), all additional spleen must be removed. Most often they are found in children and in patients with blood diseases. The additional lobe of the spleen is an innate feature and is not a pathology. But it must be differentiated with visceral lymph nodes, visualization of which is possible in most cases when they increase or change the structure.

Pathotopography (Figure 91). With small dimensions of the additional lobule of the spleen, asymptomatic flow is characteristic. Reaching large sizes, they can cause unpleasant pain, cause intestinal obstruction, make it difficult to diagnose the disease correctly and cause severe and dangerous conditions in case of torsion and necrosis of these formations. They have a diameter of up to 120 mm. They are of the same size as the spleen or even more. Most often, this pathology does not manifest itself and does not need treatment. It does not affect the quality of life in any way, therefore it is diagnosed accidentally. Most often, such abnormalities appear in the gate area of this organ. Sometimes such pathologies grow in the omentum, pancreas, and testicle. The least common additional spleen is formed in the scrotum. Their number can vary from one to hundreds throughout the abdominal cavity. Sometimes the additional spleen grows on the site of the removed. In 5/6 cases, pathology is one-lobed. The presence of an

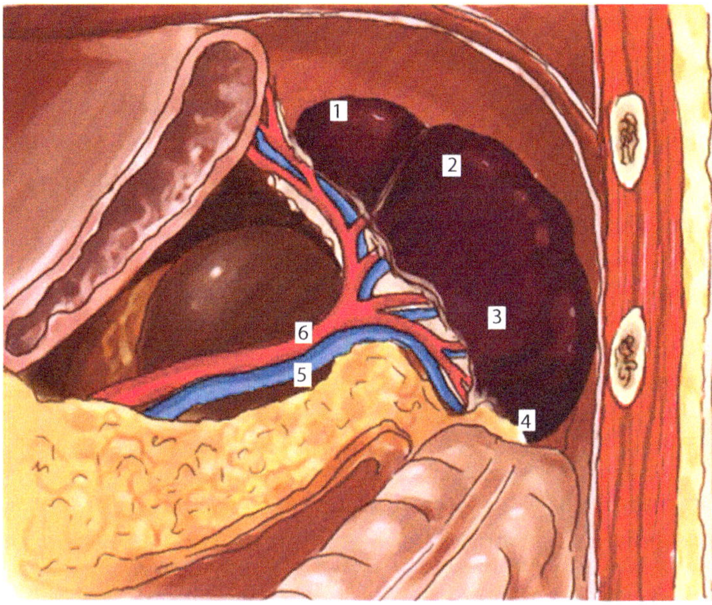

Figure 91 Additional lobe of the spleen.
1 – additional lobe of the spleen; 2 – extremitas superior; 3 – facies colica; 4 – extremitas inferior; 5 – v.lienali; 6 – a.lienalis

additional lobule increases the spleen itself. In this case, the displacement of nearby organs is observed.

Bracing or bends of the gallbladder are abnormalities in the development of the gallbladder form, leading to its deformation.

At an inflection the longitudinal axis is broken, the bubble is curtailed in the form of a cochlea, fixation by its adhesions to a duodenal intestine or a cross section of a colon is possible.

With constriction, narrowing of the gallbladder along the entire circumference or part of it occurs. Most often, constrictions and excesses are congenital in nature. In most cases, this is due to a disproportion in the growth of the gallbladder and its bed.

Deformations of the gallbladder play an important role in the violation of bile passage. The stagnant phenomena caused by this eventually lead to the development of dystrophic changes in the wall of the bladder, its contractile function. Different variants of gallbladder deformities interfere with the normal function of the organ and disrupt the motility primarily in the hypotonic type. One of the most important factors affecting the function of the hollow organ is the structure of the outlet section, the path of outflow. Congenital or acquired pathology in the cervico-ductal zone early and significantly affects the functional capacity of the entire organ. In the compensation stage, sonographic examination can be used to observe the normal contractility of the bladder or hyperkinetic dyskinesia. However, the reserves of the bladder are rapidly depleted; it becomes large and flabby. Chronic violation of outflow of bile can lead to the development of cholecystitis, stone formation. In clinical practice, it is not always possible to solve the problem; the existing deformities are congenital or acquired.

Acquired deformities, unlike innate, are diverse, sometimes bizarre. The contours of the bladder are uneven, often quite pointed protrusions are found.

For differential diagnosis, sonography is used after taking a cholagogue breakfast. If there is an inborn inflection, the unusual shape of the gallbladder is preserved, and if the constriction is due to pericholecystitis - the shape of the bladder changes.

Pathopography (Figure 92). Inflection can occur in different parts of the bladder - in the area of its body, bottom or neck. By localization during the diagnosis, specialists-gastroenterologists distinguish the inflection of the lower third of the gallbladder, upper third, bottom, wall and duct of the gallbladder. More often than other varieties, the inflection of the neck of the gallbladder is diagnosed, and the most dangerous consequences are the bend of the gallbladder in the body.

The forms taken by the gallbladder as a result of deformation are very diverse and depend on the place and degree of pathology. So, it can be an inflection of a hook-like shape, in the form of an arch or an hourglass. Moreover, there may be a double bend of the gallbladder, which

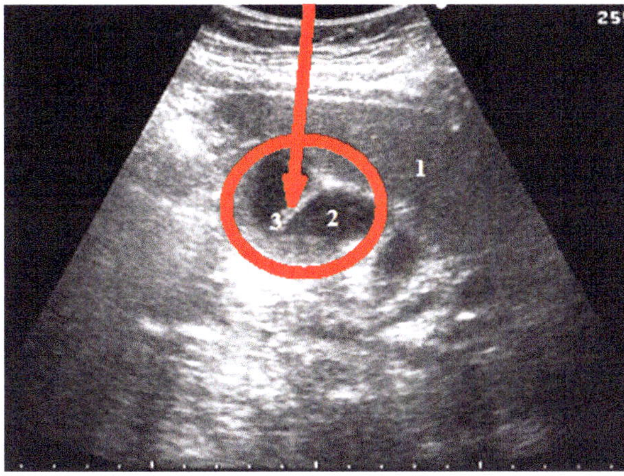

Figure 92 Anomaly of development of the gallbladder.
1 – liver; 2 – gall bladder; 3 – constriction of the gallbladder

doctors define as S-shaped and consider it the main cause of dyskinesia of bile ducts in young children.

In cases of acquired constriction, there is an acute or chronic inflammation of the gallbladder, an increase in the gallbladder or liver. Acquired inflection occurs when there is a long mesentery of the gallbladder or its complete absence, cholelithiasis.

Congenital kink is the most common anomaly that occurs in 25% of children; it is due to the development of the gall bladder during the development of the fetus.

In the first trimester, when the internal organs are placed and their subsequent differentiation, any infection, taking certain medicines, smoking or alcohol can lead to such a violation.

Cholecystitis (Figures 93, 94) is divided into 2 types:

1. Acute (calculous) - acute inflammation of the gallbladder. It refers to the number of urgent surgical diseases. Gallbladder stones and infection play a role in its development, leading to concentration, bile stasis, increased

that with phlegmonous processes the affected areas of the wall have a higher light-absorbing capacity, and with gangrenous changes the wall of the bladder becomes more "transparent". Vessels are involved in the destructive process. In the sections of the wall where intra-wall vessels can be seen, scraps of deformed vascular branches are found. With gangrenous cholecystitis, intensively shaded homogeneous, field-free fields and light zones corresponding to necrosis are seen. The picture of phlegmonous cholecystitis is also heterogeneous. With destructive forms of cholecystitis in those cases when it is still possible to see the intra-wall vessels and when inflammatory changes are not associated with too intense shading, heavy shadows are formed, along the large vessels of the fibrous layer. With continuous intensive shading, the angioarchectonics of the inflammatory process cannot be determined. In histological studies, the light zones correspond to the necrosis of the wall until the mucous layer is completely melted. Acute cholecystitis is complicated by perforation of the gallbladder wall and bile peritonitis; in the case of closure of the cystic duct and accumulation of pus in the cavity of the gallbladder – the empyema of the gallbladder; purulent cholangitis and cholangiolitis; pericholecystitis with the formation of adhesions; transition of an acute process into a chronic one. Also, the inflammatory process can pass to other organs with the development of pancreatitis, liver abscess.

2. Chronic cholecystitis. The pathogenesis of the disease is associated with impaired motor function of the gallbladder. Normal circulation of bile is broken; stasis and thickening occur. Later, the infection joins. There is an inflammatory process. With chronic cholecystitis, inflammation develops more slowly, and can gradually move from the walls of the gallbladder to the biliary tract. With prolonged flow, spikes, deformations of the bladder, fusion with adjacent organs (intestines), fistulas can form.

Cancer of the cardiac part of the stomach is a malignant formation that affects the mucous epithelium of the organ.

There are three forms of the disease:

1. painless form characterized by the presence of symptoms, but the absence of pain syndrome;

2. latent form proceeds without visible symptoms, the tumor is revealed, as a rule, suddenly, during any diagnostics or by means of palpation, when the formation has reached impressive volumes;

3. painful form. The patient is disturbed by the systematic pain in the stomach that can radiate to the lumbar region, often associated with eating. Pain can be intense, permanent, intensified when walking and it happens for a long time.

Pathotopography (Figures 95–98). A particularly complex form of cancer is a cardiac esophageal cancer. At the junction of the esophagus with the stomach, the epithelium changes in a different structure. Cancer can start from the stomach and from the esophagus (flat) epithelium, and starting from the side of the esophagus, it can be an adenocarcinoma, and not a squamous cell tumor, since its source is the dystopia of the gastric epithelium into the esophageal mucosa.

When the tumor grows into the blood vessels, gastric bleeding may occur. The consequences of cancer: anemia, reduced nutrition, cancer intoxication lead to the development of general weakness, high fatigue. The presence of any of the above symptoms is not sufficient to diagnose cancer of the stomach, thus other diseases of the stomach and digestive organs may manifest themselves. The diagnosis of "stomach cancer" is established on the basis of the biopsy data.

Polyposis of the intestine is a pathology characterized by the presence of multiple polyps in the large intestine. The polyp is the outgrowth

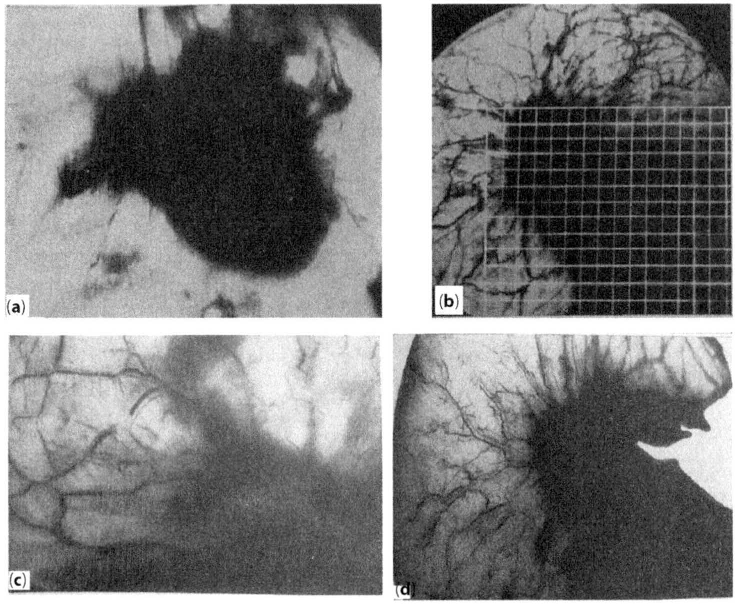

Figure 95 Planar shadow image of a cancerous focus.
a – uneven distribution of tumor infiltration in different directions; b – projection mesh, layered on the shadow image of stomach cancer; c – the advanced spread of cancer along the course of the submucosal vessel; g – tumor "clutches" around the vessels of the submucosal plexus

of the mucous membrane of the intestinal wall. Polyps of the large intestine can be single and multiple, located on a pedicle or on a wide base ("sessile"). Depending on the shape and features of the structure, different types of polyps are distinguished. Particularly, the polyps are distinguished into inflammatory (appearing on the site of inflammation), hyperplastic (the result of excessive proliferation of normal tissue) and neoplastic (growth of atypical cells). The latter can be both benign and malignant.

Pathotopography (Figure 99). When examining the leg of a polyp in transmitted light, large vessels of the submucosal layer are seen, which are directed toward the base of the polyp. These vessels are much larger in caliber than the adjacent branches, also located in the submucosa. On transillumination angiograms, it can be seen that large-sized polyps are associated with large diameter branches, and small-sized polyps are associated with small-caliber vessels. Thus, the blood supply

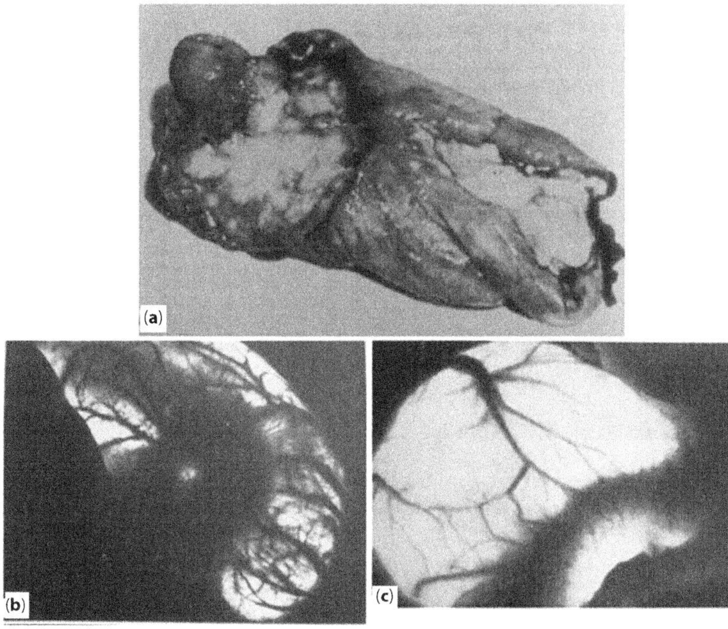

Figure 96 Saucer-like stomach cancer.
1 – macro preparation; 2 – intense ring-shaped shadow with rounded clearing in the center of the focus; 3 – radial convergence of submucous layer vessels to the central parts of the focus (b and c – transillumination angiograms)

corresponds to the mass of the tumor. Typically, polyps are located at the junction of several branches and are associated with the vessels of the submucosal plexus. Polyps are not found in those parts of the wall that are devoid of vascular branches.

The branches going to the polyp are wider than similar branches that are not related to the growth. The polyp can serve as a fixation site for several intra-wall vessels of the submucosal plexus. In inflation, these vessels arch towards the polyps. Smaller polyps do not significantly change the transillumination pattern. To the shadow images of the vessels of the submucosal plexus adjoin images of the oval form and small diameter, up to point, intensive shadow foci. Large diameter polyps are usually located along the vessel, to which adjoin.

As can be seen on the resulting angiograms, at a transmission it is possible to find out polyps of very small sizes. The general structure

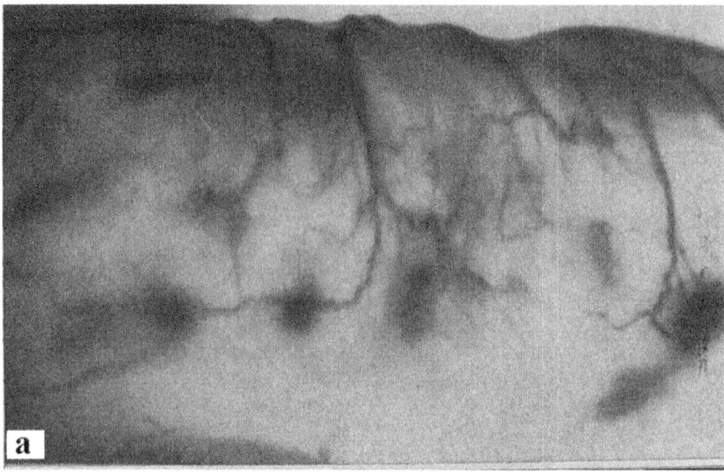

Figure 100 Chronic ulcerative colitis.

Pathotopography (Figure 100). Colitis is characterized by a tendency to ulceration of the mucosa. The pathological process does not capture the small intestine and affects only parts of the large intestine, not the entire surface. The disease manifests either in the rectum or in the sigmoid colon. Then there is a further spread of the inflammatory process. Most often the disease begins to develop gradually, with diarrhea, which is caused by the development of extensive inflammation in the intestinal mucosa. Against this background, the reabsorption of sodium and water stops. Blood appears due to the fact that ulcers form on the shell, forming a loose connective tissue, penetrated by the vascular network. The symptomatology has the property of decreasing, and then gaining momentum again.

Changes in chronic ulcerative colitis that seem diffuse during examination, in transmitted light, create a non-uniform pattern in various parts of the affected bowel. Along with the relatively homogeneous shading in some departments, enlightenment is defined in others. Local focal shadows and their relationship to intra-wall vessels are of greatest interest. They correspond to more pronounced inflammatory infiltration and are located in the zone of branching of the direct arteries. Rounded or oval focal shadows and intense shadow veils of irregular shape are formed here. Features of the shadow pattern indicate the influence of the vascular component on the formation of an inflammatory focus in chronic colitis.

With transillumination, folds of the mucous membrane are revealed – gastric fields, intestinal crypts. With a giant hypertrophic gastritis, persistent changes in the relief of the mucous membrane may disappear as the inflation increases. Dilation of thickened folds in polypoid protrusions indicates that they are associated with contracture of the muscular layer of the mucous membrane. By illumination it is possible to define a granular relief of a mucous membrane at a papillary gastritis, a zone of focal atrophy of it, and recognize a lymphomatous gastritis.

Retroperitoneal Space

Liquid formation is a cavity filled with liquid contents delimited by capsule and tissue from the bulk of the organ. It has a diverse form, more often – round, as a rule, clearly delineated, in the lumen of liquid formations, various structures are often revealed – partitions, inclusions, amorphous masses.

Liquid formations of the retroperitoneal space are inflammatory infiltrates, cysts, abscesses, hematomas in the lysis stage, cystadenomas, cystadenocarcinomas. The source of these pathological processes is mainly the organs of the retroperitoneal space – the pancreas, the descending and horizontal parts of the duodenum, the ascending and descending colon, the adrenal glands, the kidneys, ureters, large vessels, nerves, lymphatic vessels and fatty tissue.

Complications are associated, as a rule, with the nature of the pathological process. They can manifest in the form of compression of surrounding organs (cysts, hematomas, cystadenocarcinomas); the appearance of sites of inflammation in healthy tissues (abscesses); spreading to neighboring areas, development of secondary osteomyelitis (abscesses, cystadenocarcinomas); bleeding, perforation (cysts).

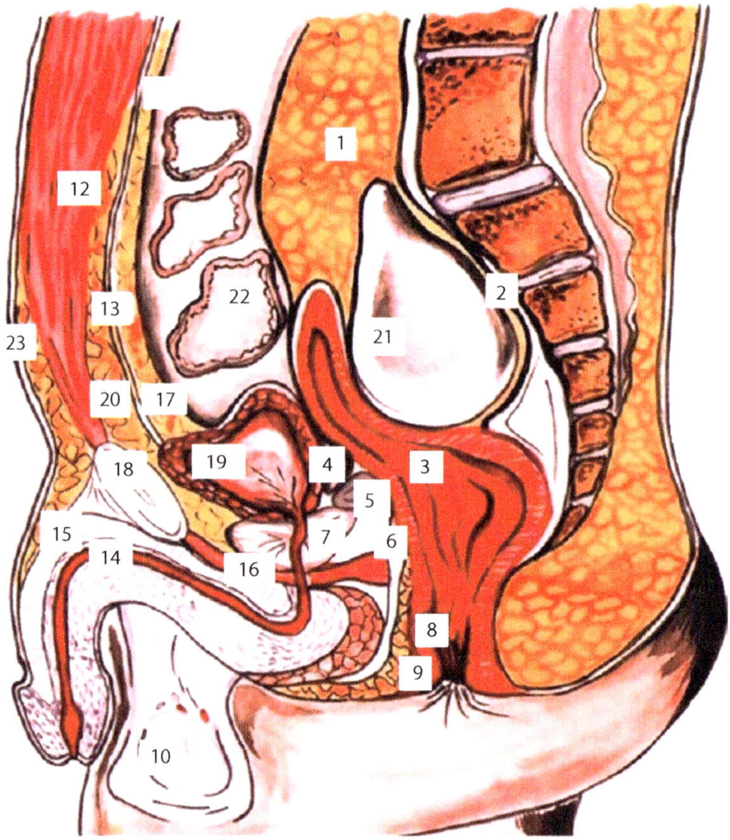

Figure 101 Sagittal male pelvis.
1 – paniculus pararectalis; 2 – a parietal leaf of the pelvic fascia; 3 – rectum; 4-recessus rectovesicale; 5 – vesicular seminalis; 6 -aponeurosis peritoneoperineus; 7 – prostata; 8 – m.sphincter ani internus; 9 – m. sphincter ani externus; 10 – testis; 11 – peritoneum; 12 – m. rectus abdominis et fascia transversus; 13 – fascia precystica; 14 – urethra; 15 – corpus cavernosum penis; 16-diaphragma urogenitale; 17 – panniculus preperitonealis; 18 – simphisis; 19 – vesica urinaria; 20 – panniculus precysticus; 21 – liquid formation in retroperitoneal space; 22 – lemniscus intestine; 23 – paries abdominalis anterior

Pathotopography (Figure 101). This figure shows an abnormality of the topography of the abdominal and pelvic organs, caused by the accumulation of a significant amount of fluid in the retroperitoneal space at the level of the sacrum. Bowel loops, bladder, and rectum are shifted towards the anterior abdominal wall and compressed, as can be judged from the considerable deformation of the contours in the direction of flattening and narrowing of the lumens of hollow organs.

The pancreas cyst is a pathological cavity that has arisen in pancreatic tissue containing a pancreatic secret and tissue detritus. For the formation of the pancreas cyst, the following conditions should be observed: damage of the parenchyma of the organ, difficulty in the outflow of pancreatic secretions, and local microcirculatory disturbance.

Pancreatic cysts are divided into congenital (true) and acquired (false, pseudocysts). Congenital cysts can be congenital, dermoid and cystic pancreofibrosis. Acquired cysts (postpancreatic retention, parasitic, posttraumatic, neoplastic) occur as a result of obturation of large or small excretory ducts of the gland and secret stagnation in them. After necrosis or inflammation of the pancreas, the formation of cysts in the obstruction of the ducts is facilitated by sclerotic changes that prevent the secretion of secrets through the lymphatic pathways. Above the site of the duct obturation there is a sacciform formation.

Pathotopography (Figures 102, 103). Primary cysts often have small dimensions. With cystic fibrosis, a pathological, viscous secretion is found that is rich in glycoproteins. This secret stagnates in the ducts and obturates them. Exocrine tissue is atrophied and replaced by

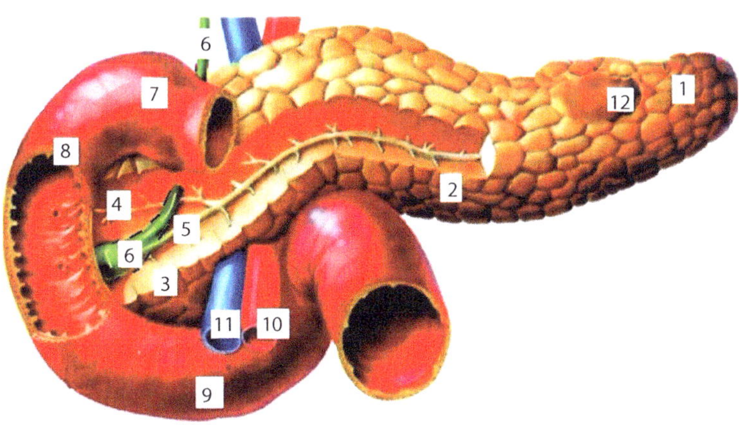

Figure 102 Cyst of pancreas.
1 – cauda pancreatic; 2 – corpus pancreatic; 3 – processus uncinatus; 4 – ductus pancreaticus accesorius; 5 – ductus pancreaticus; 6 – ductus choledochus; 7 – pars horisontalis duodeni superior; 8 – pars descendens duodeni;9 - pars horisontalis duodeni inferior; 10 – a. mesenterica superior; 11 – v. mesenterica superior; 12 – cyst

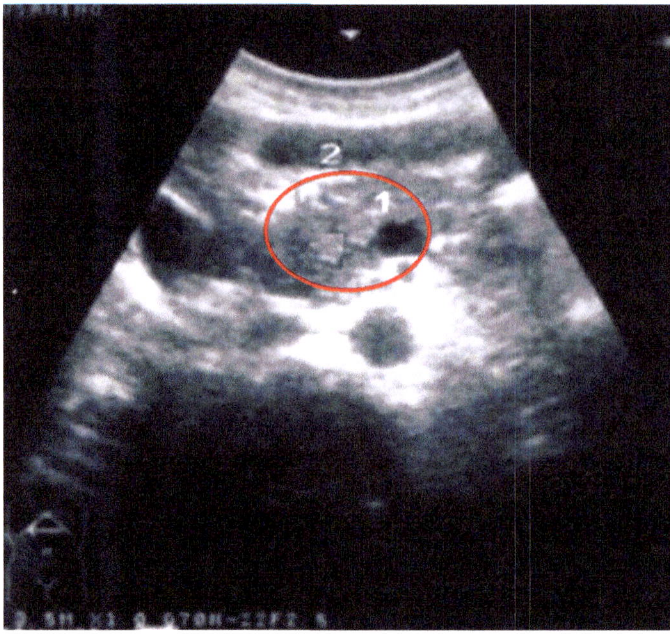

Figure 104 Chronic pancreatitis.
1 – the altered structure of the parenchyma of the pancreas; 2 – liver

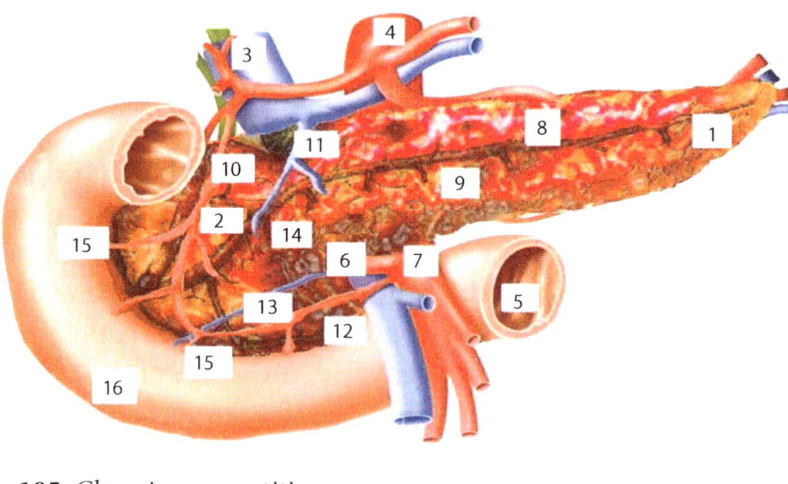

Figure 105 Chronic pancreatitis.
1 – caudapancreatis; 2 – caput pancreatis; 3 – v. cava inferior; 4 – aorta; 5 – flexura duodenojejunalis; 6 - v. mesenterica superior; 7-a. mesenterica superior; 8 – rr. glandulares; 9 – corpus pancreatic, 10 – a. pancreaticoduodenalis superior; 11 – v. pancreaticoduodenalis superior; 12 – a. pancreaticoduodenalis inferior; 13 – v.pancreaticoduodenalis inferior; 14 – processusuncinatus; 15 – rr. intestinalis; 16 - duodenum

are cicatricial changes, obscuration and disturbance of the patency of the ducts, the size of the pancreas decreases, it wrinkles and acquires a dense, cartilaginous consistency. In the ducts, protein masses are deposited. In the interstitial tissue there are inflammatory changes, around the ducts is formed fibrous tissue. In obturation of small ducts, their expansion occurs, there are rounded cavities surrounded by a cubic epithelium. Also, stones can be found inside the ducts. Due to the expansion of the ducts, retention cysts are formed. The parenchyma of the gland is replaced by peri- and intralobular fibrosis, after which the islets are destroyed. The development of fibrous tissue around the nerve endings causes significant pain.

In chronic pancreatitis, the following complications can occur: severe diabetes mellitus, splenic vein thrombosis, development of scar-inflammatory stenosis of the pancreatic duct and large duodenal papilla, internal bleeding due to the ulceration or perforation of hollow organs, infections and infectious complications (abscess, parapancreatitis, phlegmon of retroperitoneal tissue , inflammation of the biliary tract). Against the background of long-term pancreatitis, the secondary development of pancreatic cancer is possible.

The kidney cyst is a benign, rounded saccate neoplasm limited by a connective tissue capsule filled with transparent lemon content.

The following types of cysts are distinguished: simple and complex (the delineation of these categories of cysts is particularly important in connection with the high probability of degeneration into cancer of complex cysts); hereditary and acquired; single and multiple; two-sided and one-sided. By localization: they can be located under the capsule of the kidney, in the thickness of the renal parenchyma, in the region of the pelvis and the vessels of the kidney (parapelvic). Depending on the risk of development in the cyst the classification Bosniak 1986 is used. The higher the category, the higher the risk of malignancy.

Pathotopography (Figure 106). In larger cysts (more than 5 cm), more often as a result of trauma, a rupture can occur, in which the

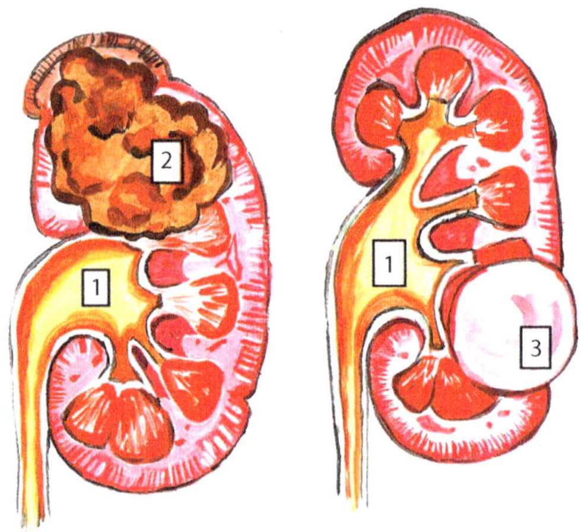

Figure 106 Renal neoplasms.
1 – the renal pelvis; 2 – Tumor of the kidney; 3 – kidney cyst

contents of the cyst are emptied into the renal tubular system or into the retroperitoneal space.

If the cyst is of sufficient size or located in such a way that the pelvic or ureteral compression occurs, then the outflow of urine occurs, which subsequently leads to hydronephrosis (expansion of the renal and pelvic system). The fact of hydronephrosis existence contributes to chronic recurrent infection, stone formation and the development of renal failure.

Uncomplicated kidney cysts, and more likely single ones, rarely lead to kidney failure. Despite the fact that the kidney cysts are often asymptomatic, it must be remembered that there is a risk of developing a malignant tumor – renal cell carcinoma.

Renal tumors are pathological proliferation of kidney tissue, consisting of qualitatively changed cells.

Depending on the nature of growth, benign and malignant kidney tumors are distinguished.

The causes of kidney tumors can be hormonal, radiation, chemical factors.

Benign tumors of the kidneys are less common than malignant. The average age of detection of kidney neoplasms is 70 years, and in men, the kidney tumor develops 2 times more often. Kidney tumors in children, from the point of view of the sex of the child, occur with equal frequency. It is characteristic that malignant tumors in children in most cases are of a mixed nature and are referred to as Wilms tumor.

Pathotopography (Figures 106, 107). The clinical picture of kidney tumors is diverse. In some cases, tumors for a long time are not accompanied by subjective sensations. The diagnosis is established by examining the patient for another disease, most often in connection with the appearance of metastases in the lungs, bones, etc.

A large group consists of tumors of the renal pelvis, although they are many times less common than kidney tumors. In benign tumors of the pelvis the most common is a transitional cell papilloma, which can be

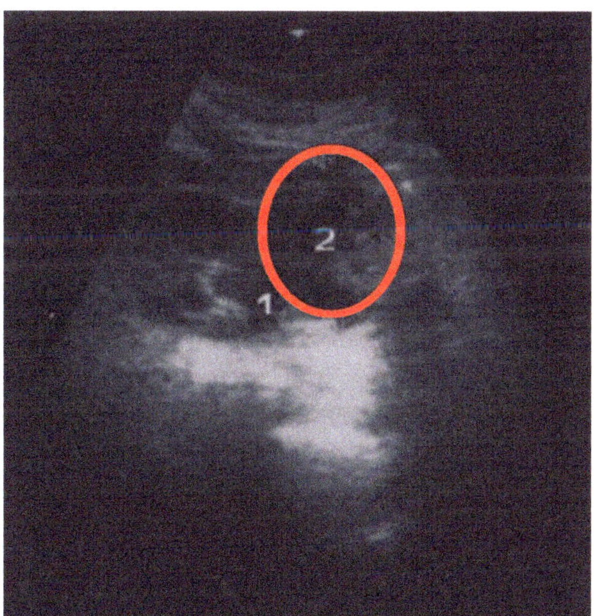

Figure 107 Tumor of the kidney.
1 – the kidney; 2 – formation (tumor) of the kidney

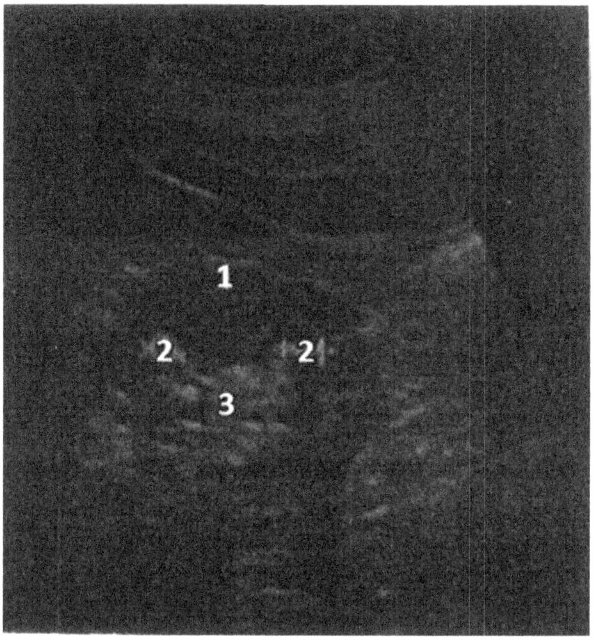

Figure 109 Urolithiasis disease.
1 – the kidney; 2 – concrement in the renal pelvis; 3 – renal pelvis

of tissues progresses, nerve and muscle fibers can become atrophic, and the ureter tonus decreases.

Ultrasound examination can be successfully used to diagnose bladder concrements and the intramural ureter. On the echogram, the stones are defined as clearly contoured single or multiple echopositive formations located on the posterior wall of the bladder or in the ureter.

About the Author

Z. M. Seagal – the Honored Scientist of the Russian Federation and the Udmurt Republic, Honorary Academician of the Izhevsk State Medical Academy, Head of the Department of Operative Surgery and Topographic Anatomy, Doctor of Medical Sciences, Professor.

Also of Interest

By the same author:

Topographical and Pathotopographical Atlas of the Head and Neck, by Z. M. Seagal, ISBN 9781119459736. Filled with detailed pictures, this atlas details the topographical and pathotopographical anatomy of the head and neck, as a useful reference for medical professionals and students alike. *NOW AVAILABLE!*

Ultrasonic Topographical and Pathotopographical Anatomy: A Color Atlas, by Z. M. Seagal and O. V. Surnina, ISBN 9781119223573. Using ultrasonic technology to create full-color detailed pictures, this atlas details the topographical and pathotopographical anatomy of the human body, as a useful reference for medical professionals and students alike. *NOW AVAILABLE!*

Check out these other titles from Scrivener Publishing:

Compendium of Biophysics, by Andrey B. Rubin, ISBN 9781119160250. The most thorough coverage of biophysics available, in a handy, easy-to-read volume, perfect as a reference for experienced engineers or as a textbook for the novice. *NOW AVAILABLE!*

Fundamentals of Biophysics, by Andrey B. Rubin, ISBN 9781118842454. The most up-to-date and thorough textbook on the fundamentals of biophysics, for the student, professor, or engineer. *NOW AVAILABLE!*

Printed and bound by CPI Group (UK) Ltd, Croydon, CR0 4YY
17/09/2026
14964243-0003